The 17 Day Diet

BREAKTHROUGH EDITION

· ·

DR. MIKE MORENO

SIMON & SCHUSTER

NEW YORK   LONDON   TORONTO   SYDNEY   NEW DELHI

Note to Readers: This publication is intended to provide helpful and informative material. It is not intended to diagnose, treat, cure, or prevent any health problem or condition, nor is it intended to replace the advice of a physician. No action should be taken solely on the contents of this book. Always consult your physician or qualified health-care professional on any matters regarding your health and before adopting any suggestions in this book or drawing inferences from it.

The author and publisher specifically disclaim all responsibility for any liability, loss or risk, personal or otherwise, which is incurred as a consequence, directly or indirectly, from the use or application of any contents of this book.

Any and all product names referenced within this book are the trademarks of their respective owners. None of these owners have sponsored, authorized, endorsed, or approved this book. Always read all information provided by the manufacturers' product labels before using their products. The author and publisher are not responsible for claims made by manufacturers about their products. The statements made in this book have not been evaluated by the Food and Drug Administration.

Simon & Schuster
1230 Avenue of the Americas
New York, NY 10020

First Free Press hardcover edition March 2011. First Simon & Schuster hardcover Breakthrough Edition January 2014

SIMON & SCHUSTER and colophon are registered trademarks of Simon & Schuster, Inc.

For information about special discounts for bulk purchases, please contact Simon & Schuster Special Sales at 1-866-506-1949 or business@simonandschuster.com.

The Simon & Schuster Speakers Bureau can bring authors to your live event. For more information or to book an event, contact the Simon & Schuster Speakers Bureau at 1-866-248-3049 or visit our website at www.simonspeakers.com.

Interior design by Maura Rosenthal

Manufactured in the United States of America

10   9   8   7   6   5   4   3   2   1

Library of Congress Cataloging-in-Publication Data

Moreno, Mike.
   [17 day diet]
   The 17 day diet breakthrough edition / Dr. Mike Moreno.—Simon & Schuster hardcover edition.
       pages   cm
   Revision of: 17 day diet.—New York : Free Press, 2011.
   1. Reducing diets.   2. Weight loss.   I. Title.   II. Title: Seventeen day diet breakthrough edition.
   RM222.2.M5683   2014
   613.2'5—dc23   2013035561

ISBN 978-1-4767-5607-3
ISBN 978-1-4767-5608-0 (ebook)

I dedicate this book to my family and friends who have supported me and my dreams, but, most important, to my mother and father who always encouraged and supported me. They placed a big emphasis on education, and instilled in me the importance of hard work and helping others. I would also like to thank my patients for providing me with the motivation to think outside the box, in hopes of making this world a healthier, happier place.

CONTENTS

ACKNOWLEDGMENTS

I feel a deep sense of gratitude to Maggie Greenwood-Robinson. Without her persistence and endless hours of dedication to this project, the book you are holding might not have been written. I'd also like to thank the many people involved in putting the program and its support materials together.

My hope is that this book will help make the world a healthier and happier place.

It's never too late to be fit and fabulous!

INTRODUCTION

Breakthrough Weight Loss

I am a guy who likes to fix things, which is probably why I chose the field of medicine and became a doctor. We doctors like to fix people; we like to make them feel better, get well, be healthier, and enjoy long, productive lives. We have even tried to fix Medicare for people, but we have not been very good at it.

Which brings me to the book you are holding in your hands: *The 17 Day Diet Breakthrough Edition*. This book is my attempt over the last two years to fix and tweak the original 17 Day Diet so that you can lose weight even faster, keep it off longer, and stay healthy and fit well into your golden years.

Before I tell you why it is a "breakthrough," let me explain why I have become so passionate about updating this book: Habits, including dietary ones, can be hard to break. For example, an estimated 144 million American adults—representing 66.3 percent of the adult population—are overweight or obese, according to the American Heart Association. Among other things, obesity and being overweight put them at increased risk for shortened lives, and, as a healer, this concerns me greatly.

The list of problems caused by obesity gets longer and longer every year, and I see most of these on a daily basis in my medical practice. Take a peek:

Heart disease and stroke. If you let yourself get very overweight, this elevates levels of artery-clogging LDL cholesterol in your body, which leads to the buildup of plaque in arteries feeding the heart or brain. Your risk of heart attack and stroke under these conditions multiplies by 10, compared to someone without a serious weight problem. Once this sort of heart damage has taken place, it can be a rapid downhill course, right to the graveyard.

High blood pressure. With excess fat on and in your body, the volume of blood your heart must pump will swell. This places pressure on your artery walls, heightening your risk of heart attack, stroke, and kidney disease.

Type 2 diabetes. This form of diabetes is on a steep rise, and the main reason is being overweight and obesity. When someone is very heavy, the body can't use insulin properly to normalize blood sugar levels. Excess blood sugar does damage our organs, arteries, nerves, and blood vessels. The consequences can be heart attack, stroke, kidney failure, neuropathy (loss of feeling in limbs), and blindness.

Joint disease. Wouldn't you like to be limber and mobile your entire life? If so, keep your weight under control. The more body weight you tote around, the greater stress you place on your joints. This greatly elevates your risk of getting osteoarthritis in your knees, hips, and lower back.

Cancer. Most people never make the connection, but being overweight increases your risk of cancer. The main cancers affected are of the colon, breast, endometrium, esophagus, pancreas, kidney, thyroid, and gall bladder.

Breathing problems. Ever heard of sleep apnea? It occurs when you stop breathing during sleep, followed by an abrupt gasp for air and loud snoring—a heart attack risk factor.

To go on with the list, it is also known that women who are overweight are more at risk for infertility, and pregnant women who are overweight have babies who are also more prone to develop hypertension, diabetes, and heart diseases.

And there are gallstones and gout, not to mention emotional disorders such as depression and social embarrassment and ridicule as a result of being overweight or obese.

I'm probably listing stuff you've already heard a hundred times. In fact, I bet you can recite the list yourself. And I know that these conditions generally don't motivate people to lose weight.

Honestly, what does motivate people to diet is the desire to look, and feel, more attractive. In other words, we slim down mostly out of vanity. That's not to say you can do things for more than one reason. I exercise regularly myself, and my diet is deliberately based on the 17 Day Diet. The rationales are multiple: My diet gives me energy and ensures I sleep well. Oh, somewhere in the mix looms a certain concern for my health: I don't want to die of heart disease, diabetes, cancer, or any of the diseases linked to being overweight. I feel that the aims of well-being and a pleasing appearance aren't at odds with each other. But of course, the bottom line is that I want to look good.

And you want to look good, too, or you wouldn't be reading this book. That mighty motivation leads to a lower risk of all those nasty diseases I listed above. Vanity—well, let's just say it's the health motivator of motivators.

Unfortunately, many of my colleagues in the medical profession have accepted that being overweight and obesity are here to stay. I do not share their opinion. Losing weight and bringing about a complete end to obesity may appear difficult considering how pervasive food is, but it is not impossible. If everyone put forth their best effort, we can definitely counter this. I have personally seen thousands of people, who used to habitually wolf down bags of cookies frequently, quit the habit in one go. And if someone has decided to lose weight for good but is unsure or having difficulty in doing it, we doctors should be able to help them if they come to us. *The 17 Day Diet Breakthrough Edition* is one more way in which I would like to help you.

The Breakthroughs

By definition, a "breakthrough" is an important discovery. Breakthroughs have been happening since ancient times, and they have altered our most basic beliefs. People used to think the earth was flat, until Columbus's voyages proved that the earth is round. The once nearly universal notion that disease had a supernatural cause was abandoned when Louis Pasteur discovered that microorganisms in the air were the perpetrators of many diseases. In 1940, a man named George Stibitz, working at his kitchen table, built the first computer that could perform sophisticated mathematical calculations. This device led to the development of the personal computer (PC), which hit the marketplace in the late 1970s. Today, the computer, the Internet, and social media have revolutionized every aspect of life, including personal relationships.

Similar breakthroughs have occurred in the field of nutrition. In the late 19th century, millers used to get rid of that ugly brown stuff that coats rice and wheat, so people could enjoy pure, refined flour in light, airy breads and pastries. The discarded roughage was fed to livestock. A century later, nutritional experts lambasted white flour and rice, after discovering that the discarded bran can protect health and save lives. For decades, the B vitamin choline was relegated to the status of a second-class, unnecessary nutrient until recent studies discovered that it is essential for a healthy liver and brain. Getting adequate choline from the once much-maligned egg yolk and other foods may even help guard against cancer and heart disease. And once upon a time, federal law limited what vitamin makers could claim about whether a supplement could cure or prevent a disease. But with so many positive breakthroughs into the benefits of supplements in improving health, the FDA, in 2000, granted supplement manufacturers the right to state that their products can improve the structure or function of the body. The FDA allows such statements as: "calcium builds strong bones," "fiber maintains bowel regularity," "antioxidants maintain cell integrity," "help maintain heart and vascular health," and so forth.

And so, in tweaking and updating this edition, I've included several diet-related breakthroughs that will help you lose weight and keep it off more effectively. Here they are:

Eat, and See Spot Melt

For decades, doctors and dieters alike have lived under the assumption that there is no such thing as "spot reduction." By that, I mean the removal of fat from selected areas of the body, through diet and exercise (not liposuction, which is surgical spot reduction). As a doctor, I am always asked how can fat be trimmed from the waist, hips, or thighs, and patients are very specific about desiring this. Is it possible to lose inches only in the areas you would like to? Yes, and it can be done with certain foods that I call "Contour Foods"—foods that have been scientifically proven to take fat off your abs, thighs, and all over your body. And guess what else? These foods happen to be very healthy. They are foods everyone should be eating, every day. So, in addition to improving your waistline and other parts of your body, you will be improving your health.

Exercise, and See Spot Melt More

And, for the first time ever, you will be introduced to the exclusive 17 Day Diet Spot Reduction Workout. I discovered a batch of research showing that certain methods of exercising, namely targeted high-repetition moves, will indeed burn fat from troublesome areas and change your overall shape, regardless of your genetics. There was not a workout per se in the original book. But since exercise is so important to fast and lasting weight loss, I wanted to make sure that the new book had a breakthrough workout component, but not just any 'ole component, rather one that would really target ugly fat, incinerate it, and get you in the best possible shape—as soon as possible!

The Transitional Day Fast

I want your weight loss with *The 17 Day Diet Breakthrough Edition* to be even faster (but still healthy), so I created an optional fast for you to follow every 17 days—if you want to. But don't worry, this fast does not mean going 24 hours without food. Not at all. You get to enjoy some delicious fasting drinks that include known fat-burning ingredients. Fasting is no longer the wicked stepmother of dieting. Increasingly, it is being scientifically recognized as a safe, healthy, and fast way to take off weight. Although fasting has been around for centuries, new ways of fasting make it a true breakthrough. My optional fast is a dietary breakthrough.

Breakthrough Supplements That Encourage Weight Loss

Natural weight-loss supplements have been on the market for more than 20 years. Until only recently, most were bogus, with false claims and hype. Now there has been enormous, credible research in this area, and there is good news from the lab: Several supplements have been found to work pretty darn well, especially when paired with the right diet and exercise program. I've scoured the supplement research the past two years to come up with breakthrough products that would complement the 17 Day Diet, and I explain the virtues of those supplements here and how to use them on the program.

Everything Works Together

The above breakthroughs work together with the powerful original features of the 17 Day Diet to further accelerate your results. Those features include the breakthrough fat-burning benefits of probiotics, such as yogurt and other cultured foods, cleansing vegetables that help your digestive system better process calories, and friendly fats that work their own weight-control magic. The diet still emphasizes a protein-carbohydrate balance designed for rapid weight loss. Of the three macronutrients (carbohydrates, protein, and dietary fat), protein has the greatest fat-burning and weigh-control effect. If you overeat calories from carbs and dietary fat, those calories will be packed away as body fat. Protein, on the other hand, is not likely to accumulate as fat. I'm not saying you can stuff yourself with protein. I am saying you should eat more protein in the proper portions from lean meat, poultry, or fish instead of pigging out on extra carbs or fat to satisfy your hunger or cravings. What's more, the diet itself is still organized around 4 cycles that keep your body constantly guessing so that you rarely plateau. And with your faster metabolism, you'll burn off calories and body fat around the clock!

A Personal Message to My Readers, New and Old

The 17 Day Diet sold well over a million copies, and for that, I am eternally grateful to have affected so many lives. If you are among that million, you are probably wondering what's in this new book for me? To that I would say, "plenty." Yes, you'll read much of the same advice, because it's foundational information that makes the diet work, but as our cars need tune-ups, maybe you need to tune up your basic knowledge of the diet. You're also graduating to the next class of the diet where you'll gain breakthrough knowledge of how to control your weight. You're going to learn a lot more that can help you, from the science of Contour Foods and spot reduction exercise to the value of fasting and supplementing.

And, you'll reap the benefits of 50 new recipes, and brand-new meal plans that include those recipes! I am a doctor who can stand the heat in the kitchen. Cooking has always been appealing to me because I can explore and expand my knowledge of different foods. I like to cook because I love the satisfaction when I've finished and tasted it, plus I like to show other people how to cook in a healthy fashion. Thus, many of these new dishes are straight from my own kitchen.

Now, maybe there are some of you out there who followed the original diet, but gained some weight back. Maybe you got pregnant after losing weight on the original diet, and need to take that post-baby weight off. Maybe you just got lax with your eating, and a lot of your weight crept back on. Ah, I see a few of you out there. Well, this breakthrough version of the 17 Day Diet can give you a totally fresh start. Once you're back on board, your body will start burning body fat once again, and you'll see results in the first days. Don't feel guilty about getting off it, just climb back on and go from there. This is your starting line in the race to get trim and healthy.

Getting back in a shape takes some fundamental commitments. If you don't exercise, start the 17 Minute Spot Reduction Workout. If you eat too much junk, start adding more fruits, vegetables, protein, and Contour Foods to your diet. Think about how this book can help you get and stay healthy for life, and make that your ultimate resolution.

And if you are brand new to the 17 Day Diet concepts, welcome! I can't wait for you to get started. You'll be amazed at the fast results you'll get the very first 17 days. You won't feel hungry, you won't be craving foods, and the weight loss you'll experience from the get-go will inspire you to keep going on down to your goal weight. I bet that at the next party you attend, your friends will gather around you, asking, "How did you lose so much weight? You look fantastic!" Simply tell them, *The 17 Day Diet Breakthrough Edition."*

So now, as you go forward with the 17 Day Diet expect to experience many great benefits:

- The loss of up to a pound a day, particularly in the first 17 days
- Steady, satisfying weight loss, right now to your goal weight
- Toned, firm hips and thighs
- A flatter belly
- Improved body shape
- Measureable loss of inches
- Satisfaction after eating, with reduced hunger and cravings
- No diet boredom

- Better overall level of fitness and energy
- Greater self-confidence
- Positive feelings about yourself and your body
- Improved health

The 17 Day Diet Breakthrough Edition is geared for rapid, healthy weight loss and targeted bodyshaping. It is easy to follow, easy to live with, and provides satisfying results. Enjoy this enhanced version. Embrace it, whether you've followed the original or not. Get trim and fit in the process—you could be as much as 17 pounds lighter after the first cycle of the diet. So . . . if that sounds good to you, and if you're ready to start—or restart—turn the page and let's do it!

PART ONE

. . . .

The 17 Day Diet Breakthrough

1

Just Give Me 17 Days

I can personally sum up the 17 Day Diet in two words: fast results.

And now, with the introduction of *The 17 Day Diet Breakthrough Edition*, I can say *faster results*. I've tuned up the original diet with some new science, new tips, and new techniques that will help you to lose up to a pound a day in the first 17 days and to keep losing steadily after that.

Since the publication of the *The 17 Day Diet*, testimonials of rapid, effective, and lasting weight losses have poured into my office and have been posted on blogs and websites. The response has been downright amazing and overwhelming—much of it unsolicited, and from practically every corner of the world. Add these to my own weight-loss patients, and there are now millions of people who have discovered a diet they love and can live with.

Here are just a handful of typical comments that have come to me from my patients and other dieters—some in person, others by e-mail, and still others by Internet posts in chatrooms:

• • • • • • • •

I lost 70 pounds on the 17 Day Diet—almost half a person. This is the first diet I've ever been successful on. I did it with my 17 year-old-son, too; he needed to slim down after football season and he lost 15 pounds. Doing it together was a bonding experience, and I feel like it changed my family's health.

• • • • • • • •

I found out through a manager of a clothing store about your diet. She had lost 80 pounds and looked great. And, she is keeping it off! After finding out about the 17 Day Diet and how balanced it is, I immediately ran out and bought the book. My husband and I started on it a week ago. I've lost

8 pounds and he has lost 9 pounds—and that is in the first week. We are thrilled and wanted to email you about how well the diet is working.

· · · · · · · ·

I am very short (5 feet), but I weighed too much for my height: 154. I found out about the 17 Day Diet so I picked up a copy of the book. I am a native of Thailand, and I found the diet very easy to follow according to the way we eat here. I now weigh 105, which is perfect for my size. Best of all, I feel so well, with lots of energy and very good health. I changed my entire eating behavior towards more nutritious foods, and I am very happy with my life at this new, slimmer weight. Thank you, Dr. Mike.

· · · · · · · ·

I am currently on Cycle 1. My roommate and I started this diet 8 days ago. I have lost 8 pounds in my first week. I am so excited! And my pants feel a little baggy. I'm still hoping to lose another 17 pounds or so on this diet. Hopefully, the rest of cycle 1 and all of cycle 2 will get me there.

· · · · · · · ·

I followed the diet through each cycle. I lost 11 pounds in the first 17 days and over the remaining course of the diet I lost a total of 27 pounds. I had learned so much from Dr. Moreno's diet and method. I eat more often, in smaller amounts, and I have kept it off.

· · · · · · · ·

I started the 17 Day Diet in mid-September. I reached my first goal of a 20-pound weight loss by Thanksgiving. After the holiday season, I went back to the first phase and continued to a 37-pound loss by the end of June. I have continued to follow the basics of the diet and have learned to take control of the food I am eating. I feel great! I also dropped 4 sizes. People are constantly asking how I did it, and of course I refer them to the 17 Day Diet.

· · · · · · · ·

This diet has been a life changer for me. I feel great every single day. I have more energy and I feel less bloated. I have lost 12 pounds, and I'm only on Phase 1! I have tried a number of diets before this one and I have never lost this much, this fast.

· · · · · · · ·

I am a woman in her fifties, and I have had weight issues most of my life. I have reduced and regained a few times. Recently I saw Dr. Mike on *The Doctors,* and I believe it was a life changing moment. I lost 10 pounds in the first three days! Then I was hooked because I felt better, and weight was coming off without counting calories! I dieted when I was in my twenties and it was never this easy! Really. I got so excited that I started telling people about the program. I have now completed the four 17 day cycles and lost 39 pounds.

You'll hear more testimonials like these later in the book in sections called "I Broke Through!"

Even More Rapid Results

Depending on your weight when you start out and your metabolism, you might lose up to 10 to 12 pounds in the first 17 days. Of course, the further you are from your ideal weight, the more you'll initially lose. And, with this new, revised version of the diet, I've got some tricks up my white-coat sleeves to help you lose even faster.

Let's not kid each other: When you start a diet, you want to see results right away, in how you look and in how you feel. That's because our society is geared toward the immediate; we want things and we want them now. The same is true of weight loss. We get impatient when the pounds don't come off fast enough. It seems much easier to give up than to go on.

This diet is designed to produce quick results, not because it starves you down to size, but because its carefully designed balance of food and exercise adjusts your body metabolically, so that you burn fat, day in and day out.

Also important: The weight-reduction portion of this diet is limited to just 17 days at a time, so you aren't demoralized by the thought of endless months of dieting.

Nor are you apt to plateau as you might do on other diets. The 17 Day Diet keeps your body and metabolism guessing. I call this *body confusion*. With each 17 Day Cycle, and my new Transitional Day Fast between cycles, you're changing your calorie count and the foods you eat. By varying these things, you prevent your body from adapting. The scale is less likely to get stuck. The added bonus: You'll never get bored; it's fun watching those pounds melt off. So, confusion is good!

At the end of 17 days, you'll go on to a second 17 Day Cycle, then a third, and finally enter the weight-stabilization cycle of the diet, in which you get to eat a greater variety of foods, including your favorite foods *within reason*. (I don't want you to get too chummy with the all-you-can-eat buffet again.)

I already know what you're thinking: Is it possible to shed pounds swiftly yet safely? If done right, without sacrificing good nutrition, the answer is yes.

Despite what many nutritionists have preached for years, rapid weight-loss diets can be healthy if done correctly, and can work wonders, reducing pounds and inches in just days. Research published in the *International Journal of Behavioral Medicine* suggests that the faster you take weight off, the longer you keep it off. That's a reason for dieters everywhere to rejoice. Plus, if you're too embarrassed by a recent weight spike or have just gained an embarrassing eight pounds after a holiday weekend or an ice-cream binge, this diet can get you back on track fast.

The 17 Day Diet thus gives your body the perfect jump start, the kind of quick drop in weight that gives you a powerful mental boost. My whole focus is to get you thin as soon as I can. When I do, just think: You'll no longer have to move around hauling the equivalent of two 40-pound bags of cement. The button on your jeans will no longer pop out and ping off the wall. You'll no longer have to wear plus-sized clothing with expandable waistlines. This diet will make you slim, healthy, and curvy, and I won't make you chomp on celery sticks, or follow some hardcore exercise regimen used by the Navy Seals.

However, you do have to accept that this won't be a pleasure diet. You've got to stop eating unhealthy crap. You've got to eat vegetables, fruit, and lean meat. I'm not going to ask you to probe your inner eater and uncover emotional reasons that you're fat. I am going to ask you to keep your portions down, cut your intake of fatty, sugary, salty foods, and move your butt. You won't be faint with hunger or found in the kitchen at midnight, feeding on Froot Loops and tubes of cookie dough. You can do this, because anyone can do anything for 17 days.

MISTER M.D., CAN YOU PLEASE TELL ME ?

But Won't a Lot of the Weight I Lose Be Water Weight?

Yes! And that's awesome, because water is weight, too. Never dismiss those extra pounds as only water weight; this is a self-defeating attitude. Cosmetically, water weight can hide fat loss and be particularly frustrating. Healthwise, fluid retention can put a strain on your heart. When your body holds water, this means there's more water in your blood. Your heart has to work harder to pump all that extra volume. Once all that excess fluid has disappeared, so will your bloat and puffiness. You'll start looking visibly thinner in three or four days. And, chances are, you'll feel much lighter and be more motivated to watch what you eat.

The beauty of this program is that you won't be discouraged or bored by the prospect of staying on a diet for what seems like forever. It can yield results that will stand the test of time just as well as those long-term diets that emphasize depressingly slow incremental drops in weight. You'll love the fact that in 7, 10, or 17 days, you'll be slimmer. And chances are, you'll feel a lot lighter and have an absurd amount of energy.

The 17 Day Diet is doable and easy—unlike so many other diets, which are slightly less complicated than the checklist for a shuttle launch.

SCIENCE SAYS: Slow Isn't Necessarily Better

Conventional wisdom says that rapid weight loss leads to rapid weight regain. A new generation of science, however, shows that slow isn't necessarily better.

Shape Up the Fast Way. A 2010 study from the University of Florida suggests that the key to long-term weight loss and maintenance is to lose weight quickly, not gradually. Among 262 obese middle-aged women, fast weight losers were those who shed more than 2 pounds a week. Compared to more gradual losers, fast weight losers lost more weight overall, maintained their weight loss longer and were less likely to put weight back on. The findings were published in the *International Journal of Behavioral Medicine*.

Trim Belly Fat. We pack on two forms of belly fat. One type collects around internal organs, known as *visceral fat*. This type of fat raises blood pressure and cholesterol levels, and increases the risk of diabetes, Alzheimer's, and even some cancers. Visceral fat is far more sinister than fat elsewhere in the body.

The other type sits just under the skin and is known as *subcutaneous abdominal fat*. It causes a hard-to-get-rid-of belly pouch. In a Finnish study published in the *International Journal of Obesity and Related Metabolic Disorders*, a rapid weight loss diet followed for 6 weeks trimmed visceral abdominal fat by 25 percent and abdominal subcutaneous fat by 16 percent. The 17 Day Diet now emphasizes specific Contour Foods that target belly fat, so say goodbye to that spare tire and hello to flat abs.

So, can you give me just 17 days?

If you can, congratulations! You won't be disappointed.

What Lies Ahead?

So, what is *The 17 Day Diet Breakthrough Edition*? I'll go into depth in the next few chapters, but, in a very quick summary, it is a fun, fantastic way of eating designed to take off weight quickly. It's based on some very simple principles, one of which is eating foods that favor fat burning, help change your body contours, and are friendly to your digestive system.

I want to emphasize that excess weight is always a sign of nutritional and metabolic imbalance. Contrary to popular assumption, it's not strictly a question of how much exercise you do or how much food you eat. Rather, it's also a question of what types of foods are eaten, and how they are digested, assimilated, and metabolized. If any of these components of good nutrition are compromised, then the body will not be adequately nourished at the cellular level, metabolic function will be impaired, and toxins will accumulate. Thus, to lose weight fast we need to optimize digestion and metabolism. That's what the 17 Day Diet does.

Trust me, you'll love the rapid loss of a few pounds so much that you'll decide to keep on going. After the first 17 days, there are another 17 days, and another: 3 total cycles and a maintenance cycle, during which you get to eat whatever the heck you want, mainly on weekends. Here's an overview:

Quick and Easy Overview of the 17 Day Diet	
Cycles	*Purpose*
Cycle 1: Accelerate (17 days)	To promote rapid weight loss by improving digestive health. It helps clear sugar from the blood to boost fat-burning and discourage fat storage.
Cycle 2: Activate (17 days)	To reset your metabolism through a strategy that involves increasing and decreasing your caloric consumption to stimulate fat burning and to help prevent plateaus.
Cycle 3: Achieve (17 days)	To develop good eating habits through the reintroduction of additional foods and move you closer to your goal weight.
Cycle 4: Arrive (ongoing)	To keep you at your goal weight through a program of eating that lets you enjoy your favorite foods on weekends, while eating healthfully during the week.
Transitional Day Fast between cycles	To coax your body into additional fat-burning between cycles in order to maintain your fast results. This tool is completely optional.

Once we're through with all the basics, I'm going to talk to you about how to follow the diet. I can't wait to show you all its wonderful components and start you on your way to looking fit and fabulous. Take it one step at a time, so that you don't feel overwhelmed.

Your Appointment with Me

I might as well take a moment here to introduce myself. I'm a family practice doctor. Under America's health-insurance system, most people go first to a doctor like me for all complaints, from infections to chronic illnesses. I love the diversity of family practice. One moment, I'm treating an 18-year-old guy with the flu; the next, a 90-year-old woman with joint pain.

I became a doctor for the reasons most people do—because I wanted to save lives, pure and simple. In my heart of hearts, I believe a doctor is so much more than a person who dispenses medication or marks off symptoms like a checklist at a sushi bar. He or she should treat the whole person. I make it a point to get to know each patient as a person before I put a stethoscope to his or her chest.

I run my office a little differently than most. Nowadays, you spend more time waiting in the examining room than you do in the waiting room. In fact, you spend more time in the examining room than the person who decorated it. It's almost like going to a restaurant and being told that, even though you have a reservation, you have to sit at the bar for a while. The only difference is that in the doctor's office, no one offers you a cocktail, and you have to wear a boxy blue paper exam gown that opens in the front.

The next time you have to wait in the examining room, do some fun things to pass the time. Glue the tongue depressors together into coasters and sell them to other patients. Or peel off all the wallpaper without disturbing any of the diplomas.

In my office, my patients don't wait forever. My patients often don't even sit on the examining table when I talk to them. I sit on the examining table and they get the comfortable chair. The butcher paper upholstering the examining table is wonderful to draw on. Sometimes I hop off the table and start drawing pictures of organs to explain things to patients.

I'm responsible for 2,000 patients, though not all in one day. Many of them are women, and 80 percent of my new patients are overweight. Most know it. One of the things I've always found interesting is that my patients often come in with a complaint of back pain, or knee pain, or just plain old fatigue. Before I can get a word out, they say, "I know it's because I'm fat." Patients are smart.

Ever since I became a doctor, I've been concerned with prevention. Prevention is the doorway to longevity. I hate shoving medications at problems that can be fixed with simple changes in lifestyle.

A good example is a patient I'll call Sharon, age 60. Sharon has type 2 diabetes. When I first started seeing her, she was taking oral diabetes medication. Once she changed to a healthier diet and started walking regularly with a friend, she was able to get off all her meds. What a triumph that was!

Then, a few years ago, Sharon came in for her regular appointment. We reviewed the results of her latest blood work. Her sugars were through the roof. Her A1C test, which reflects a patient's blood sugar over the past 90 days, was suddenly out of range.

What on earth had happened?

As we talked, Sharon told me that she no longer had a walking partner, so she had quit exercising altogether.

"I'll walk with you!" I volunteered. I couldn't bear to see her health slip. And, so, I became her walking partner. Before long, others joined us. Our walking group became affectionately known as *Walk with Your Doc* and has swelled to more than 50 people of all ages. We walk every Tuesday and Thursday morning without fail. I love it, because I thrive on helping people live full, healthy, active lives.

Of course, a huge part of prevention is weight management. You see, the death toll racked up by heart disease, high blood pressure, stroke, diabetes, and all the other fat-related diseases is scary. Studies even associate obesity with poor immune function. That makes overweight people more susceptible to infections and cancer. Obesity will kill far more Americans each year than any terrorist would dare dream of taking out.

Everybody knows this. I'm just bringing it up again to remind you that tubs of ice cream and bags full of chips are not worth shortening your life.

MISTER M.D., CAN YOU PLEASE TELL ME

Do I Have to Exercise While on the 17 Day Diet?

Yes, but I won't be asking you to sweat to golden oldies, pump it up, or feel the burn. In other words, no over exercising. Since you'll be scaling back on calories, you should do less exercising, or else you'll get too run down and sore, especially during the first two cycles. I will ask you, however, to do just 17 minutes a day of easy exercising. You'll find my exercise instructions in chapter 15: The 17 Minute Spot Reduction Workout. It will show you how to exercise in a way that provides spot shaping and spot conditioning of your body. Hey, I not only want you to lose body fat, I also want to you to reshape your body. I'll show you how in that chapter.

I should add that the 17 Day Diet has a companion exercise DVD, called the *17 Minute Workout*, which you can purchase from our website, www.the 17daydiet.com. It's cardio based and geared toward pure fat burning.

So, for now, put down this book. Do this workout, or go outside and walk around your neighborhood for 17 minutes. Then come back and pick up where you left off.

We're already in so much trouble with trans fats, cheap sugars, excess sodium, and unpronounceable additives jazzing up junk food—stuff that causes your arteries to clog like rusty pipes. With everything plaguing the American diet, I had to concentrate on creating a program that would be safe, effective, and produce quick but lasting results. People had to get the weight off, then learn how to keep it off. I didn't want to tell my patients to go on this diet or that diet because many diets are nutritionally unbalanced, hard to follow, or just don't work fast enough to keep you motivated.

Thus, the 17 Day Diet evolved. It uses the latest medical knowledge on nutrition, foods, and what the body needs for successful weight loss and good health.

Let me add here: You should check with your own physician before starting this program. Your doctor knows what's best for you. Based on my experience with my own patients, most people who have gotten out of shape over the years can follow the 17 Day Diet and do very well on it, though results can vary.

There Is More to Love about
The 17 Day Diet Breakthrough Edition

Whether you've got 10 pounds to lose or a hundred, being overweight is one of life's lesser joys. It affects every aspect of your life, maybe some things you never thought about. When you lose weight, practically everything in your life will change for the better. Let's talk about this.

The Antioxidant Advantage

If you talk to folks who have lost weight on the 17 Day Diet, you'll see that not only are they slimmer and fitter, but that their skin glows and they look practically ageless. And they may tell you that they're full of newfound energy. Why is this?

The foods you eat on the 17 Day Diet are brimming with antioxidants, which are essential to your health. When you're overweight, your fat cells become a repository for toxins from environmental pollutants, food preservatives, chemicals, and pesticides. This toxicity is why you may feel tired, be bloated, have drawn-looking skin, suffer constipation, or have joint pain or headaches, and it may be why your metabolism is so slow. Your body just can't work optimally when loaded down with toxins. Studies have in fact found that people who are overweight or obese are often dangerously low in antioxidants.

How do antioxidants help you? When you start supplying your body with antioxidant nutrients from food (and to some degree, supplements), particularly vitamins C and E, beta-carotene, and minerals like selenium and zinc, these nutrients go to work and rid fat cells of toxins. This nutritional rescue improves the way your body works, how you feel, and the efficiency of your metabolism.

Get a Healthy Bod

You're going to be focused on losing pounds and inches. Some days, you might get a little discouraged if the scale doesn't move down fast enough, even though this diet does help prevent plateaus. But there's absolutely nothing to be discouraged about. As I alluded to in the Introduction, the diet can reverse many overweight-related issues, which means that there are other wonderful things happening inside your body that won't be reflected on the scale, like your blood pressure, blood sugar, and cholesterol decreasing.

Okay, I realize that right now you might not care about these things. You just want to slip into that sexy black number hanging in your closet . . . you know, the one that used to fit years ago. However, it's important to understand that your weight and health are not separate issues. Being overweight is a symptom of being unhealthy. Focus on your weight and your health will improve—instantly. Consider what the results of various research studies say about the rather immediate effects of healthy nutrition on the body:

After 15 minutes: After the first morning of eating a healthy breakfast, your stomach's satiety signals have registered in your brain, and you feel full. The body's internal chemistry is at its most active first thing in the morning, so your breakfast is then used to the maximum.

If you eliminated processed foods (white bread, sugary cereals) for whole grains and lean proteins like egg whites, along with fresh fruit, you should feel energetic and mentally alert after just one meal.

After 3 hours: Your artery linings are able to expand sufficiently to increase blood flow to the body's tissues and organs.

After 6 hours: The HDL (happy cholesterol) in your blood perks up and starts scouring LDL (lousy cholesterol) from the blood. You can think of LDLs as delivery trucks, depositing cholesterol in blood vessels, and HDLs as garbage trucks, taking them back to the liver where they're broken down.

After 12 hours: Your body finally has an opportunity to burn the fat it has stored for energy because you've eliminated sugar. When you're eating a lot of sugar, your body is so busy processing the sugar that it doesn't have time to do its other job, which is to help the body burn fat. So guess what? The fat ends up hanging around.

After 16 hours: You get a restful night's sleep.

After 24 hours: You're 1 to 2 pounds lighter, because your body has begun to flush excess water and toxins from your system.

After 3 days: Once your body senses that it's losing weight, its blood-related numbers (cholesterol, blood pressure, blood sugar) start traveling in a healthy direction.

After 1 week: Your cholesterol levels can drop significantly. Blood levels of important disease-fighting antioxidants like vitamin C and vitamin E are higher. Your bowels are in better working order, and you should be at least 5 pounds lighter.

After 2 weeks: You'll experience healthy drops in blood pressure if you've been diagnosed with hypertension. Expect to have lost up to 10 pounds by now.

After 1 month: Nobody has to filter out chunks of fast food from your blood anymore. By now, blood levels of LDL cholesterol can fall by nearly 30 percent—a drop similar to that seen with some cholesterol-lowering drugs.

After 6 weeks: You've lost so much weight you can't buy new, smaller clothes fast enough. Yes, you should have lost quite a bit of weight (20 pounds is not unusual), and your blood cholesterol and triglyceride levels will be substantially improved.

After 12 weeks: Many significant health numbers—cholesterol, triglycerides (fat in the blood), blood pressure, glucose, and insulin—should begin to, if not completely, normalize.

After 6 months: You'll feel healthier because your body will be retaining more vitamins and minerals. Because you reduced your sugar intake significantly over this period, insulin production will have normalized. Thus, your risk of developing type 2 diabetes is reduced, as this can be linked to a larger intake of sugar. Your energy levels have improved dramatically because your body has gone through a detoxing process. You've probably reached your goal. The hardest work is over, and now it's time to learn how to eat to maintain your newly slender silhouette.

Pretty amazing what a good diet can do, right? Don't you want all of this? Be brutally honest here: If you really want something you'll find a way to get it. So, if you find yourself saying, "I didn't have time to prepare healthy food," let me ask you this: would you have found time if your life depended on it? Well, it does.

GET SKINNY SHORTCUT

Posture. Stand up straight. Not only does slouching make your belly protrude, but it gives your core muscles an undeserved break. Standing erect, with the stomach held in, encourages the abs to work and can make you look slimmer naturally—and in an instant.

Get Sexy

When you're fit and in shape, you're much more datable. In one survey of 554 undergrads, researchers found that overweight women were less likely to date than their peers. What's more, you're marriage material if you're thin. Research shows that overweight women are significantly less likely to marry than are women of average weight, particularly if they were overweight as young adults.

Losing weight can do wonders for your sex life, too. Duke University researchers did a study of 187 extremely obese adults, who were asked about their sex lives before and after they lost weight. It turned out the proportion of women who did not feel sexually attractive fell from 68 percent before they began a weight loss program to 26 percent a year later. There were similar decreases in the percentages of women who didn't want to be seen naked, had little sexual drive, avoided sexual encounters, had difficulty with sexual performance, or didn't enjoy sex. Among men, sex improved in most of the categories, but the improvements were less dramatic, probably because there are a lot more appearance-related pressures on women.

The romantic world revolves around physical appearance. If you want a love life with great sex, lose the weight.

Get Richer

Get in shape and you can improve your financial shape, too. It's considerably more expensive to be unfit than it is to be fit, mainly because you're sicker more often and you pay higher medical bills. People who are overweight, and particularly those who are obese, are significantly more likely to have expensive-to-treat diseases like diabetes, heart disease, and cancer.

And, while I'm at it, did you know your employment prospects will improve after you lose weight? It's true! People with weight problems sometimes don't get hired. In the job market, appearance counts for a lot. Employers think fat people are lazy, incompetent, slow moving, and might have poor attendance. Studies have shown that fat people are paid less than employees of average weight.

I hate fat discrimination. It's wrong. But this is the world we live in. It's not going to change anytime soon, so get over it. Lose weight and you won't have to deal with it.

Thin people look better, and, like it or not, get paid more. If you're trim and healthy, you don't have an absentee problem. You might even be more productive on the job. All of this helps your earning potential. So, if you want to live well and make your mortgage or rent payment, get those pounds off.

If my message seems too in your face, I apologize for the delivery, but not for the content. I'm speaking out because I care. I just want you to get healthy and enjoy your life to the fullest.

LEAN 17: Are You Ready to Be a Total Hottie or Hunk?

Take this quiz to see if you are ready to go on the 17 Day Diet. A successful and healthy weight loss requires the right frame of mind. Circle the answer that best describes your level of commitment.

1. When I think about starting the 17 Day Diet, I feel excited.
   A. Yes   B. Somewhat   C. Unsure   D. Not at all

2. I feel that weight loss and fitness are very important.
   A. Yes   B. Somewhat   C. Unsure   D. Not at all

3. I am determined to eat more healthfully.
   A. Yes   B. Somewhat   C. Unsure   D. Not at all

4. I want to look better and feel sexier.
   A. Yes   B. Somewhat   C. Unsure   D. Not at all

5. I am willing to follow the food plans in this book.
   A. Yes   B. Somewhat   C. Unsure   D. Not at all

6. I will eat more fruits and vegetables.
   A. Yes   B. Somewhat   C. Unsure   D. Not at all

7. I will give up soft drinks, candy, and other sweets while following this diet.
   A. Yes   B. Somewhat   C. Unsure   D. Not at all

8. I will scale back on my alcohol intake.
   A. Yes   B. Somewhat   C. Unsure   D. Not at all

9. I will prepare more meals at home and eat out less frequently.
   A. Yes   B. Somewhat   C. Unsure   D. Not at all

10. I will increase my water intake.
    A. Yes   B. Somewhat   C. Unsure   D. Not at all

11. I am willing to cut back on starchy foods like white bread, pasta, and sugary breakfast cereals.
    A. Yes   B. Somewhat   C. Unsure   D. Not at all

12. I feel confident that I can stick to this plan for at least 17 days.
    A. Yes   B. Somewhat   C. Unsure   D. Not at all

13. I will eat at least 3 meals and 1 snack a day.

A. Yes   B. Somewhat   C. Unsure   D. Not at all

14. I will not make excuses to sabotage myself.

A. Yes   B. Somewhat   C. Unsure   D. Not at all

15. I can commit to exercising for at least 17 minutes a day.

A. Yes   B. Somewhat   C. Unsure   D. Not at all

16. I want to change my eating and health habits for life.

A. Yes   B. Somewhat   C. Unsure   D. Not at all

17. I understand how diet, obesity, and chronic illnesses are linked.

A. Yes   B. Somewhat   C. Unsure   D. Not at all

Scoring: Give yourself a 3 for each A answer; a 2 for each B answer; a 1 for each C answer; and 0 for each D answer. Add up your score.

0 to 17 points: Immediately reevaluate your commitment to improving your health. If you don't act decisively now, serious health problems are on the horizon.

18 to 26 points: Go back over your answers and see what you need to shore up. You may be taking some unnecessary risks with your health and should make an extra effort to change.

27 to 42 points: Reexamine your desire to go on the 17 Day Diet. What improvements can you make to boost your score? You need just a little bit more determination and commitment to be thinner and healthier.

43 to 51 points: You're ready to start the 17 Day Diet and enjoy success—congratulations!

You must believe that you can do this. It doesn't matter how often you have failed in the past; your past does not equal your future. What matters now is focusing on what you want, identifying what you need to get it, and taking action. Your health and happiness are important, so stand strong.

Review

- The 17 Day Diet is a rapid weight loss plan designed to produce satisfying, lasting weight loss.

- Most people can expect to lose up to 10 to 15 pounds during the first 17 days.

- Rapid weight loss plans have been shown in research to be effective in helping people keep their weight off.

- Contour foods will help change your shape for the better.

- The 17 Day Diet works by improving digestive and metabolic health.

- The 17 Day Diet is organized into 4 cycles, each working together to help your body reach its ideal weight and stabilize there.

- Stay upbeat and positive. No matter what you weigh right now, stop beating yourself up over it. So much in your life can change for the better: your figure, health, relationships, financial stability, and more.

2

Burn, Baby, Burn

ere's the part of the book in which I talk about how the 17 Day Diet works. Don't worry. I won't lapse into any mind-numbing doctor speak. You know, medical terms that sound scarier than the disease, like cephalalgia (headache) or pneumonitis (lung inflammation). Most people have no idea what their doctors are saying. They could be giving them the latest medical research or the recipe for chocolate cheesecake in Latin. They couldn't tell.

I make a real effort to explain things in everyday terms. Sometimes, it's hard. I used to try to explain blood tests to patients in five minutes. It finally dawned on me that it took me eight years to understand this stuff, so I can't expect anyone to comprehend it during one office visit. You don't need to study medicine to understand what doctors say anyway; just watch *House* and *The Doctors*.

Back to the topic of dieting: I will add Rita's story here. If the subject of weight loss came up in conversation, she'd walk away. About 25 pounds overweight, Rita was deep-down scared that she could get heavier if she didn't do something, but she just wasn't ready to confront the issue head on. The idea of dieting and taking weight off slowly was frustrating, so she kept putting it off. But the 17 Day Diet appealed to her. It sounded doable and quick—it is. Rita decided to give it a try.

Here's what she said, "I can't believe how well the diet works. I lost 10 pounds the first 17 days, and I feel so energetic. What gives? How does it work?"

Basically, Rita was hooked (in a positive way) and has used the diet to get to her goal and stay there. She stayed motivated.

I explained to Rita that for a diet and exercise program to be successful, it must be safe, easy to follow, and easy to stick to. It must have a certain balance of nutrients to activate fat burning. It must generate results in a reasonable period of time. And it must help initiate a pattern of healthy habits that leads to lifelong weight control. The 17 Day Diet can help you accomplish all of this and more. What follows is a careful look at the elements that make this diet work.

What Do You Get to Eat on the 17 Day Diet?

First, let me say that nutrition is confusing, even for doctors. Everything is either good or bad for you. And that can change from moment to moment each time a new bit of research is unveiled. Broccoli may double your life span this week, but next week it might be the end of you.

Several years ago, blueberries became the fruit of choice, touted as the answer for everything from rejuvenating your brain to inhibiting the growth of cancer cells. Now, they're being added to cosmetics. If they can prevent your brain from aging, why not put them in a skin cream? Maybe blueberries can stop wrinkles, too.

I think you have to be living under a rock not to know that lean proteins, fruits, vegetables, and small amounts of grains are naturally good for you, and that some will even help change your shape for the better, like my Contour Foods. The 17 Day Diet is based on those foods. That's one reason why the diet isn't a fad; it's based on really healthy foods, the stuff we should all be eating anyway, but aren't.

With these wonderful foods, we get the body to store the good (health-building nutrients) and expel the bad (fat and toxins) by retraining your digestive system and your metabolism.

Many long and informative books have been written about nutrition and how it works in the body. For the purpose of this book, I'll explain what you need to know about the nutrients your body needs to lose weight, and I'll do it in the clearest, most basic terms.

Enjoy Plenty of Protein

The 17 Day Diet is generous in protein. However, I don't mean 27 eggs and 18 strips of bacon washed down with the drippings. I mean lean foods such as chicken, fish, lean meats, and other protein-rich foods.

Protein is a powerful fat torcher for seven reasons:

1. Digesting protein takes more energy (calories) than digesting carbs or fat does; thus, your body burns a few extra calories after eating protein.

2. Including ample protein in your diet spurs one of your body's fat-burning mechanisms: the production of the hormone glucagon. Glucagon signals your body to move dietary fat into your bloodstream and use it for energy rather than store it.

3. Consuming enough protein helps you preserve lean muscle mass that might otherwise be sacrificed on a rapid weight loss diet. Of course, the more lean muscle you have, the more calories you burn, even at rest.

4. Most protein foods, especially fish, are Contour Foods that research has shown trims belly fat.

5. Eating protein helps keep your blood sugar on an even keel, so you don't get the shakes or drops in energy.

6. Having enough protein in your diet boosts your metabolism, and it does this by stepping up the action of your thyroid gland. (One of the main duties of the thyroid is to regulate metabolism.)

7. Including protein with meals helps tame your appetite so that you don't stuff yourself.

Venture into Vegetables

If you haven't eaten vegetables since you were 11, let's spend a second on this "I hate vegetables" thing.

You hate all vegetables? There isn't one you like, no matter how it's prepared? If you eliminate all vegetables from your diet, you're giving up some very important nutrients and really narrowing your food options. Vegetables are loaded with fiber, vitamins, minerals, and antioxidants. Shunning them is a bad idea. Why not learn to prepare them with herbs and spices to satisfy your taste?

Pardon my assumption, but I think you, like thousands of other people I've talked to, believe that to lose weight, you have to subsist on carrot and celery sticks. But the old carry-around-some-celery-sticks-to-munch-on mentality is gone forever. Aren't you relieved?

There are hundreds of different vegetables you can eat, even if you have to hide them in soups or spaghetti sauce. And you can pretty much eat your way through a couple of bushels without gaining any weight. If you want to change your body and get leaner, stronger and healthier, you have to eat vegetables. A March 1999 study conducted by the Energy Metabolism Laboratory at Tufts University found that the dieters who ate the widest variety of vegetables had the least amount of body fat. You need to eat vegetables if you want to get thin. Vegetables = thin. No vegetables = flabby.

Many of my patients have actually acquired a taste for lettuce, spinach, cucumbers, and all sorts of veggies. Some of them have even turned themselves into health nuts who only dip their forks into the salad dressing to really slash caloric intake.

There are more benefits. Eat more vegetables and you will:

- Bubble with energy all day.

- Improve your digestion and elimination, because veggies are high in fiber. High-fiber foods control appetite and help prevent excess calories from being stored as fat.

- Help your body boot out toxins that are slowing down your metabolism.

- Have glowing skin. Your skin loves vitamins, minerals, and antioxidants, and you get most of those nutrients from veggies.

- Help prevent major killers like cancer and heart disease, because veggies are rich in disease-fighting antioxidants.

So yes, you heard me: Eat your vegetables!

Forego High-Sugar Fruits

Fruit may seem like a great diet food because it's naturally low in calories and contains no fat, but still you have to be careful with fruit. A bunch of fruits, namely, pineapple, very ripe bananas, and other tropical fruits are loaded in sugar, and they don't help with fat loss very well when eaten in excess. Too much sugar from any source can convert into thigh-padding pounds.

I'm not going to ask you to shun all fruit. Just be moderate in how much you eat—two servings a day only. On the first two cycles of the

17 Day Diet, you'll stick to berries, apples, oranges, and grapefruit, which are lower in sugar. Plus, several fruits on the diet are Contour Foods that will improve your shape. By eating like this, a fruit tooth will replace the sweet one that rules your mouth.

Curb the Carbs

Carbohydrates are energy foods. Without them, you'd get fuzzy headed, cranky, and very tired, and no one will want to be around you. The low-carb diet craze deemed all carbs evil and fattening. People abandoned all forms of fruit, rice, and pasta and ate mostly protein. The problem is, you can only eat so much protein and fat before you start to get nauseated by it.

Yet, not all carbs are the same. There are bad ones—stuff that is made mostly of sugar or is overrefined like white bread, white rice, and white pasta. Sugar and sweets are the worst. Consider this: We are eating over twelve times the amount of sugar our great-grandparents consumed. That's nearly 150 pounds of sugar down the hatch of each person in the United States each year. Let me help you visualize this: Go to the supermarket and buy 150 one-pound bags of sugar. (I wonder how many carts you'll need!) Then unload them in your kitchen. Betcha there's no room in your pantry! Really get a visual here. Most of us have no idea that we're wolfing down so much sugar. Much of it is hidden away, in processed, packaged foods we eat, as well as in beverages.

Depending on which cycle you are in on the 17 Day Diet, you get to eat good carbs: fruit, vegetables, whole grains—anything that hasn't been stripped of its nutrition.

So, the type of carbs you eat is important. So is the amount. You can go overboard on carbs, even the good kind, and this can be devastating to your natural metabolic processes. Therefore, the 17 Day Diet is low to moderate in carbohydrates.

Many people are walking around completely unaware that they may be carbohydrate sensitive. When you are carbohydrate sensitive, your body can no longer burn fat effectively, and a good deal of the carbo-hydrates you eat are packed away as fat. Carbohydrate sensitivity occurs when:

- You habitually eat too much sugar and refined carbohydrates (crackers, cookies, bagels, white pasta, white bread, sugary cereals and desserts, white rice, and white bread). Unfortunately, this sensitivity increases with age. It can also lead to insulin resistance, a condition just shy of type 2 diabetes. In insulin resistance, cells don't recognize glucose anymore, so glucose is barred from entering cells for energy. Your blood sugar tends to rise, you are more fatigued, and you gain more weight mostly around your waist and chest area.

- You suffer from chronic stress. Our bodies react to stress chemically. They jack up cortisol, a hormone secreted from our adrenal glands, which prepares us to handle the stress. However, if we stay under stress, cortisol hangs around, and it floods our bloodstream with too much glucose and insulin. The result is insulin resistance. To your physiology, being under chronic stress is the same as if you ate cake all day long.

- You're a woman. While men burn carbohydrates for energy, women tend to store them as fat. This is especially true as women age. Menopausal women are more susceptible. They don't have enough estrogen to counteract cortisol and its tendency to make the body store fat. Chalk it up to female biology.

CHECK UP: Are You Carbohydrate Sensitive?

Read the statements below and circle "yes" or "no," depending on which response fits you best.

1.	I crave carbohydrates and sugary foods much of the time.	Yes	No
2.	I have been overweight for much of my life and have struggled to lose weight.	Yes	No
3.	I am a woman and over forty.	Yes	No
4.	I suffer from chronic or bouts of depression and compulsive overeating.	Yes	No
5.	I sometimes suffer from nervousness, irritability.	Yes	No
6.	When I eat sugar, I get tired and groggy, and I don't think as clearly.	Yes	No
7.	I reach for carbohydrates over protein most or all of the time.	Yes	No

8. My diet consists of a lot of processed foods like white
   bread, pastas, sweets, or sugary cereals.   Yes   No

9. I don't exercise very much or at all.   Yes   No

Natural and unprocessed carbs are found on the 17 Day Diet in the vegetables and fruits allowed you. By Cycle 3, you'll get to introduce other carbs into the diet, including brown rice, oatmeal, whole grains, yams, potatoes, and other natural, high-fiber carbs.

Choose Fats That Burn Fat

Fat in the diet has been blamed for many modern lifestyle diseases: obesity, heart disease, cancer, diabetes, and hypertension. Not all fats are created equal, however. There are bad fats: saturated fats (the marbling in meat, butter, and other animal fats), and trans fats, a commercially manufactured fat found in processed foods, mostly.

Friendly fats are found mostly in fish, veggies, and nuts. These fats are credited with keeping your skin supple and youthful, reducing harmful levels of cholesterol, lowering high blood pressure, contributing to brain and eye development, and a host of other health benefits, almost akin to a panacea. Friendly fats also promote weight loss because they keep you feeling fuller for a longer period of time. This keeps you from taking in too many calories. And, some friendly fats are Contour Foods that can help reduce your waistline.

Omega-3 fatty acids, found in fish, boost your metabolism. Adding some weekly servings of fish high in omega-3s (salmon, tuna, mackerel, or sardines), while cutting back calories, helped overweight people lose more weight than just cutting calories alone, according to a study published in the *American Journal of Clinical Nutrition*. The researchers concluded that the omega-3s assisted in the fat-burning process. If you don't like fish, take 3 grams of fish oil supplements daily.

I Did It the 17 Day Way!   Barbara

My husband and I have been married 11 years and have been trying to lose weight and be healthy most of our marriage. Both of us have always battled with our weight. When I was younger I was smaller and a little healthier but my husband has always been big. But that all changed last October. My mother-in-law is a nurse who works for a hospital. She also battles with her weight. One of her coworkers told her about your 17 Day Diet that she and her husband had been on. They were having good results, so my mother-in-law went on the diet and got great results. Naturally, my husband wanted to try it, but I didn't. I was tired of trying to lose weight only to gain it back. However, I had a scare while on vacation that changed my mind.

We went to Destin, Florida, with our family. I tend to be hypoglycemic, so I had eaten a big breakfast one morning. While walking on the beach, I started shaking and almost passed out. It took me several hours to start feeling better. I realized that I had eaten too many carbs during the big breakfast. Then my husband wanted to go parasailing but thought he was too big. All of this was very frustrating. After we got back from Destin, we decided to try the 17 Day Diet. That was on October 8, 2011. It was the day that changed our lives forever.

We know that this plan has saved our lives. I have lost 126 pounds and my husband has lost over 200. We don't know the total amount for him because we couldn't find a scale that would weigh him until he had been on the diet about 2 months and lost two pant sizes. We are pretty sure that in April of 2011 he was about 500 pounds. He is now 223 pounds. He was wearing a 50 in pants and 5x in his shirt. Now he is a 34 in pants and an XL in shirt. My highest weight was 340 and I wore a size 32. I had lost some weight down to 300 but was starting to put it back on. Now I weigh 174 and wear a 12–14. We have been maintaining for several months.

The most wonderful part of all this is the people that have been inspired by us to also make a change in their lives. I got your e-mail from the ladies at my mother's church in Lebanon, Tennessee. They got in touch with you, and you sent cookbooks for a Ladies Day they were having. I spoke that day and told them our journey of weight lost and better health. Those ladies stared the diet and lost lots of weight. Most of our church members have been on the diet. So have our friends, family, and co-workers. I could go on with how we have been impacted by your diet. But the main thing we want to say is "thank you" for taking the time to care about your patients and to put together a plan to save their lives and ours.

Vitamins from Food

You're better off getting your vitamins from food. The body absorbs them more easily, and you'll just feel healthier. Required by your body in tiny amounts, vitamins play important roles in the metabolism of carbohydrates, proteins, and fats. The vitamins you need daily are found in *The 17 Day Diet Breakthrough Edition* as follows:

- *Vitamin A:* Green leafy vegetables, carrots, yams, fruits, and eggs.
- *Vitamin B-complex:* Protein foods, whole grains, legumes, fruits, and vegetables.
- *Vitamin C:* Fruits and vegetables.
- *Vitamin D:* Low-fat dairy foods, fish.
- *Vitamin E:* Whole grains, green leafy vegetables, and eggs.

Mighty Minerals

Minerals are among the heaviest substances ever, second only to Orson Welles. But, of course, minerals don't make you heavy. They help you get thin, especially calcium, which may speed up the rate at which your body burns fat.

Like vitamins, minerals are central in metabolism. However, there's one major difference between the two nutrients: Minerals are the actual building material of bodily structures, namely bone, cartilage, and teeth. Minerals make these things strong. While vitamins help manufacture these structures, they do not become part of the structures themselves.

The minerals you need daily are found in the 17 Day Diet as follows:

- *Iron:* Meats, poultry, eggs, green leafy vegetables, and fruits.

- *Calcium:* Yogurt, salmon, green leafy vegetables, and broccoli.

- *Copper:* Meats, shellfish.

- *Magnesium:* Meats.

- *Phosphorus:* Meats, poultry, fish.

- *Potassium:* Fruits and vegetables.

- *Selenium:* Whole grains, fish, and eggs.

- *Zinc:* Shellfish, meats, whole grains, and vegetables.

The Benefits of Bugs

Not the kind you swat, spray, or stomp, but the friendly bacteria called *probiotics* that live in your intestinal tract (hereafter referred to as your *gut*). You have a hundred trillion bacteria in your gut—ten times the number of cells—across three hundred to five hundred different species, and two hundred of these species can be lethal. This makes us more microbe than man. So, naturally, you want more of the good bacteria in your gut, since it helps keep the bad in check.

There are actually two processes going on here. One is that the good bacteria help your intestinal wall erect a blockade against the bad bacteria. The second is the good bacteria are like hostage negotiators you have seen on television. They talk to the bad bacteria to keep them from starting a fight. The bad bacteria know the good guys mean business, so they drop their weapons and wave white flags.

The good guys do even more: Probiotics may help people lose weight, because accumulating evidence points to obesity being partially related to an imbalance of bacteria in the gut. This is a true breakthrough discovery, and it may change the way we treat obesity.

Scientists are still exploring why, but many believe that people with a certain makeup of gut bacteria may get more calories from their food and, therefore, gain weight more easily than folks with a different collection of bugs. If you have a set of very, very efficient bacteria, they're going to gobble every last bit of energy (calories) from what you eat. Manipulating these bacteria by diet or medications, you'd change how many calories you absorb. This may eventually become one important approach to fighting obesity.

On the 17 Day Diet, you'll enjoy foods that contain probiotics. These foods help your body digest foods and extract calories. Some types of probiotic foods include yogurt, kefir, miso, and tempeh.

Fluid Assets

While following the 17 Day Diet, you should drink eight 8-ounce glasses of pure water daily. Drinking this amount of water is essential to weight loss.

First, it just takes up so much space in your tummy that you don't feel like eating anything else.

Second, water also helps your body metabolize stored fat. Here's how this all works: It starts with your kidneys; they need water to help flush stuff out of your body. If there's not enough water, your kidneys go on a forced work stoppage. The liver then has to pinch-hit and fill in for the kidneys. This is not good, because one of the liver's primary functions is to turn stored fat into fuel for the body. If the liver is filling in for the kidneys, guess what? It doesn't have time to metabolize fat, so whoops, more fat stays in storage and weight loss stops.

Second, water is a natural detoxifier; it helps the body flush waste during weight loss. And, when you're shedding pounds, your body has a lot more waste to dump, including fat.

Surprisingly, drinking a lot of water is the best way to resolve water retention. When your body is dehydrated, it perceives this as a bodily drought and begins to hold on to every drop as a defense mechanism. Water is then stored outside the cells, causing your feet, ankles, legs, and hands to swell. The best solution for water retention is to give your body what it needs: plenty of water.

So, drink up. Before long, you'll be the skinniest person in the bathroom.

BEWARE: Negative Water

The following fluids, which I call negative water, do not count toward your must-have daily allotment of water.

Coffee*

Tea*

Diet sodas*

Regular soda

Energy drinks

Juice

Sports drinks
(Dilute with water—½ water and ½ sports drink, if you are an athlete and use these products.)

Flavored waters

Coffee and tea are allowed on the 17 Day Diet, but do not count toward your 8 glasses of water.

Special Mention Fluid: Green Tea

For added fat-loss benefits, another beverage of choice is green tea, although it is technically a negative water. Certain natural chemicals, called *catechins*, in green tea increase fat burning and stimulate thermogenesis, the calorie-burning process that occurs as a result of digesting and metabolizing food. Studies published in the *American Journal of Clinical Nutrition* showed that drinking green tea prevents the body from depositing excess body fat, burns more fat, and improves the way your body uses insulin, a fat-forming hormone. Also, the catechins in green tea can produce metabolic rises both during exercise and while at rest.

Since the initial publication of the original *17 Day Diet*, much more research about green tea has surfaced. The study that intrigued me the most was one in which researchers found that, by drinking green tea, you could burn an additional 70 calories over a 24-hour period. Okay, that might not seem like a lot, but let's pull out the calculator and do some simple math. Let's say you drink green tea and burn 70 calories a day because of it. There are 365 days in a year, so that's a total of 25,550 calories burned in a year. Divide that sum by 3,500 (the number of calories in a pound of fat), and you've burned off 7.3 pounds in one year, just by sipping tea!

The other point I'd like to make about green tea is that it contains about 10 times the amount of antioxidants as fruits and vegetables. By drinking green tea, you're taking in antioxidants that will help detox your cells and get your metabolism moving in the right direction. You may also extend your life. I read a study published in one of my favorite journals, *The Journal of the American Medical Association*, that followed 40,000 people for 11 years. (I'm not sure how you follow that many people; I have trouble following some of the faster walkers in my Walk with Your Doc group.) Anyway, the researchers found that people who drank around five cups of green tea daily were 31 percent less likely to die of heart disease and 42 percent less likely to pass away from stroke, compared to people who drank less than a cup of green tea a day.

Green tea is also one of the foods that may block angiogenesis (sorry, I have to slip one technical term in here). *Angiogenesis* refers to a process of blood vessel growth. For example, angiogenesis that builds up a blood supply to tumors that can, unfortunately, make the tumors grow. Scientists have discovered that angiogenesis does the same thing with fat tissue: It creates a blood supply to fat tissue too, so it can grow. Fat tissue and cancer feed on oxygen delivered by these new blood vessels.

There's excellent science published in the best journals that something in green tea inhibits angiogenesis. The jury is still out on this, but until we know more, I suggest drinking 3 to 4 cups of green tea per day to get all the known benefits. One trick that helps is to steep 2 teabags in one cup; that way you get the benefits of two cups in one, and you don't have to walk around all day with a teacup in your hand.

Although doctors should set an example, I confess I'm not much of a green tea drinker. If I'm having a cup, I'm probably in an Asian restaurant. I promise to do better, though, and drink more green tea.

Now, if you don't like green tea, here are some substitutes:

- Take capsules of green tea extract. (Follow the manufacturer's recommended dosage.)
- Stir matcha green tea powder into foods, such as smoothies, yogurt, or cereal. (This powder is very high in antioxidants.)
- Have coffee instead. Coffee is also permitted on the 17 Day Diet. The caffeine kicks your metabolism into high gear. Caffeine also jump-

starts the breakdown of fat in the body. I'd recommend sticking to 1 to 2 cups a day.

MISTER M.D., CAN YOU PLEASE TELL ME

Am I Allowed to Drink Alcohol on the 17 Day Diet?

I knew you'd ask that. Alcohol can actually be good for you. Major studies have concluded that moderate alcohol consumption cuts heart attack risk in half, largely because drinkers have about 15 percent higher levels of HDL cholesterol than nondrinkers, which prevents heart disease by cleansing the blood vessels of fatty buildups. Moderate alcohol means one drink a day: 5 ounces of wine, 12 ounces of beer, or 1½ ounces of hard liquor.

Although a little alcohol is good for your heart, it's not that good for your waistline. Alcohol is dehydrating and interferes with fat burning. The liver works overtime to metabolize the alcohol, so its job of burning fat gets less priority.

Once you get to Cycle 3, it's fine with me if you have one drink per day. Now, I don't recommend keeping it at your desk (at least for daytime use), but I do recommend it, especially red wine. One of my hobbies outside work is enjoying fine red wine. To pursue my passion for drinking and collecting red wine, I enjoy attending wine tastings with my friends.

Red wine is full of a natural chemical called *resveratrol* (a powerful antioxidant found in grape skin). It switches off a gene that activates certain inflammatory proteins in the bloodstream. When a foreign body, such as a toxin, shows up in your body, these proteins act like people addicted to Pinterest, the virtual pinboard. They (the proteins) pin those toxins right to your artery walls, which stimulates chronic inflammation. That's bad, because inflammation is known to cause clogged arteries, blood clots, impotence, and even heart attack or stroke. So, where does red wine fit in here? One glass a day may just help prevent these things. Cheers!

Are You an Early Eater or a Late Eater?

You are *when* you eat. Let me explain.

When I was a resident, I developed some bad eating habits, such as eating out of boxes and having lunch whenever I could grab it, like at four in the afternoon or even midnight. Now, I've learned that eating too late in the day makes losing weight harder.

In a study published in the *International Journal of Obesity*, researchers found that the later you eat your lunch, the more difficult it is to lose pounds and the higher your risk of getting diabetes. They studied 420 overweight people for 20 weeks; those who ate lunch after three lost significantly less weight than those who ate earlier in the day. Late eaters had a lower *insulin sensitivity*, meaning their bodies weren't metabolizing blood sugar well, a situation that can lead to weight gain and diabetes.

There's a lesson here: Try to eat a regular pattern of meals throughout the day, with main meals and snacks at roughly the same time throughout the day. The moral of this study is: No late lunches.

The 17 Day Diet allows you to snack between your main meals. That's a good thing. In fact, I want you to eat something every three hours. Research shows that folks who don't eat for three hours or longer have more body fat than regular snackers. If you go too long without eating, or if you skip meals, your body senses that food is scarce, so it clings to its energy reserve, which is fat. Then when you finally eat something, insulin shoots higher than normal in an effort to process the calories coming in. At that point, a fat-storing enzyme called *lipoprotein lipase* increases too, and starts packing away the newly eaten calories as fat.

Never fall prey to the myth that skipping meals will help you get skinny. Just the opposite: it will deter your efforts to burn fat, impair your appetite regulation (which might lead to bingeing), and undermine your metabolism. Eat on a regular schedule, and you'll lose weight easily.

How Much Should You Weigh?

As you begin the 17 Day Diet, have a specific weight goal in mind. In other words, shoot for a weight at which you feel you will look your best. Keep in mind that there's really no such thing as the so-called perfect weight, because we all come in a variety of body shapes, heights, and bone structures. There are, however, ideal weight ranges; there is a simple equation I tend to follow.

If you're a woman: Take 100 pounds for the first five feet of your height, and add five pounds for each extra inch to get the midpoint of what should be your ideal body weight range. Then, you need to factor in your body structure. Some people are small boned; others are big boned. If you're small boned, subtract 15 percent from the normal-frame weights; if you're large boned, add 15 percent to the normal-frame weights. For a lot of people, that's too much math. So, I did the math for you:

WOMEN		
Small-Boned Frame	*Midpoint*	*Large-Boned Frame*
5' = 85	5' = 100	5' = 115
5' 1" = 90	5' 1" = 105	5' 1" = 121
5' 2" = 94	5' 2" = 110	5' 2" = 127
5' 3" = 98	5' 3" = 115	5' 3" = 132
5' 4" = 102	5' 4" = 120	5' 4" = 137
5' 5" = 106	5' 5" = 125	5' 5" = 144
5' 6" = 110	5' 6" = 130	5' 6" = 150
5' 7" = 115	5' 7" = 135	5' 7" = 155
5' 8" = 119	5' 8" = 140	5' 8" = 161
5' 9" = 123	5' 9" = 145	5' 9" = 167
5' 10" = 128	5' 10" = 150	5' 10" = 173
5' 11" = 132	5' 11" = 155	5' 11" = 178
6' = 136	6' = 160	6' = 184

If you're a man: Take 110 pounds for the first five feet of your height, and add six pounds for each extra inch to get the midpoint of what should be your ideal body weight range. Allow for being small or large boned, as I've explained.

MEN		
Small-Boned Frame	*Midpoint*	*Large-Boned Frame*
5' = 94	5' = 110	5' = 127
5' 1" = 99	5' 1" = 116	5' 1" = 133
5' 2" = 104	5' 2" = 122	5' 2" = 140
5' 3" = 109	5' 3" = 128	5' 3" = 147
5' 4" = 114	5' 4" = 134	5' 4" = 154
5' 5" = 119	5' 5" = 140	5' 5" = 161
5' 6" = 124	5' 6" = 146	5' 6" = 168
5' 7" = 129	5' 7" = 152	5' 7" = 175
5' 8" = 134	5' 8" = 158	5' 8" = 182
5' 9" = 139	5' 9" = 164	5' 9" = 189
5' 10" = 145	5' 10" = 170	5' 10" = 196
5' 11" = 150	5' 11" = 176	5' 11" = 202
6' = 155	6' = 182	6' = 209
6' 1" = 160	6' 1" = 188	6' 1" = 216
6' 2" = 165	6' 2" = 194	6' 2" = 223
6' 3" = 170	6' 3" = 200	6' 3" = 230
6' 4" = 175	6' 4" = 206	6' 4" = 237
6' 5" = 180	6' 5" = 212	6' 5" = 244
6' 6" = 185	6' 6" = 218	6' 6" = 251

How Often Should You Weigh Yourself?

Not too many people like to weigh themselves. Doctors know this. After patients step on the scale, they think it is giving them the weight of a completely different person, like Hulk Hogan. Since we won't let them weigh naked, they tell us to subtract two pounds for their shoes, one pound for jewelry, and three pounds if it is after the Big Mac and fries they had for lunch. Some people strip off this stuff faster than a Lexus left on a city side street at midnight and step on the scale again. But doctors' scales do not lie. Patients have to accept the truth. Their bodies, without consulting them, have been converting doughnuts, pizza, and ice cream into fat.

Seriously, please let us doctors help you. Yes, usually you have to strip down to your birthday suit to let us examine you. This is something that a lot of people feel embarrassed and uncomfortable about. Unfortunately though, these feelings can stop people from talking about problems they have or letting us doctors find early signs of disease long before serious trouble sets in.

Let me reassure that we know it is tough to talk about saddle bags and love handles, but we are trained to show you respect and help you feel more comfortable. Plus, we see butts, boobs, and flab so much that we are immune to it. And very few of us doctors are anywhere near the hunky or hot bodies you see on television, in the movies, or on the pages of slick magazines. (I know for one that I am a long way short of that.) So, have no fear; let us help you get to your healthiest self. We are here to make sure that you don't diet of embarrassment.

SCIENCE SAYS: Use Your Brain to Get Buff

Medical studies have shown that visualizing yourself in the shape you want to be in can help you attain a trim, toned physique. The brain thinks very much in pictures. If you can call up a picture in your mind, you have a powerful way of making it happen. So, it's important to get the image of your ideal physique in your mind so that you can create it.

Start imagining what your life will be like as a thin, healthy person. You'll be able to play, be active, really live, and enjoy living for your family. You'll be able to shop at normal stores, not wear plus-sized clothes, and forget worrying about fitting into airplane seats. You'll no longer be a target of jokes or have people judge you. And you won't have to fear a future of diabetes, heart attack, stroke, or other weight-related health issues. All these images give your mind realistic goals to work toward.

Let's talk about scales for a moment. Your bathroom scale can be a top tool for losing weight. I know, some people say throw it out, but those people are naturally thin or possibly teach aerobics classes. They don't need a scale.

If you skirt the scale, your weight might start going up, and you won't know it. Then, when the nurse forces you at pen point to ascend the scale at your next doctor's appointment and 302 pops up, you might go into shock.

Monitoring weight using the scale will prevent that from happening. It's a great habit and one that has helped people in the National Weight Control Registry—a group of several thousand successful losers—keep their weight off. People are eligible to sign up for the registry if they have lost at least 30 pounds and have maintained their weight loss for at least a year. The registry is used by researchers to learn how people actually keep their weight off, because successful losers are like aliens from another planet. When scientists can get their hands on one, they want to study it.

Yes, other things can tell you a lot about your weight: the way your clothes fit, how winded you feel going up a flight of stairs, or how you look in the mirror. But weigh yourself too, every several days, or at least once a week, and definitely after each 17 Day Cycle.

Just resist weighing yourself dozens of times a day in hopes of a better outcome.

So, take that candy jar off your desk. It may make you less popular with your co-workers, but you're on your way to a lighter life. And that's exciting.

LEAN 17: Facts About Fat

1. The average adult has 40 billion fat cells.
2. Fat is also one of the most plentiful tissues in the body.
3. Fat tissue is not inert; it is a dynamic, complex tissue, necessary for life.
4. Girls are born with more fat cells than boys.
5. By the time you're a teenager, you will likely have all the fat cells you are ever going to have.
6. Fat expands when existing cells enlarge and when new cells are born.
7. The number of fat cells can increase, but they won't decrease.
8. When you lose weight, existing fat cells shrink.
9. Fat cells die, but your body quickly replenishes them with the same number.

10. Fat cells are bigger in obese people.

11. Fat cells come in two colors: white and brown. White is the kind that makes your jeans too tight. Brown fat is found in babies and has the ability to burn energy.

12. Fat cells, like cancer cells, and other cells in the body, feed themselves oxygen through new blood vessels created in a process known as *angiogenesis*. Researchers are studying whether certain cancer drugs can starve fat cells to stop fat expansion the same way they starve tumors.

13. When you exercise, cells produce an enzyme that tells fatty tissue to release its stores for muscles to burn.

14. The liver stores *glycogen* (the storage form of glucose) and releases it into the bloodstream when energy is needed. Once glucose runs low, the body starts to burn fat for fuel.

15. Fat cells secrete estrogen, and excess estrogen is involved in the progression of certain cancers, including breast cancer.

16. Body fat accumulates from head to toe and comes off the same way.

17. Body fat is like a ski suit: It provides insulation against the cold. A downside of getting thin is that you might shiver more often.

Review

- On the 17 Day Diet, you eat healthy foods: lean proteins, vegetables, low-sugar fruits, natural carbs, probiotics, and friendly fats. These foods work together to improve your digestion and metabolism.

- The 17 Day Diet supplies the nutrients you need for good health.

- The 17 Day Diet limits carbs somewhat, because many people are *carbohydrate sensitive*, a condition that interferes with weight loss.

- Drinking water is vital for weight loss; so is drinking green tea.

- You do not skip meals or eat late lunches on the 17 Day Diet.

- Know your goal weight, and do not be afraid of the scale.

Contour Foods:
Nutritional Spot Reduction

I'm going to tippy-toe through some rather controversial territory here: spot reduction. For your entire dieting life, you've probably heard that you can't spot reduce, right? Well, it turns out that the statement that there's no such thing as spot reduction isn't entirely true. There are certain foods and nutrients that have been scientifically proven to spot reduce troublesome body parts, such as the tummy, thighs, and hips. Those foods and nutrients are included in *The 17 Day Diet Breakthrough Edition*.

Let me elaborate on what I call "Contour Foods." Science has, thankfully, identified foods that can truly change your shape. If you understand how to use these foods, then you do not need surgical liposuction. You need nutritional liposuction. It is an amazing breakthrough, and most dieters are unaware of this. So, let's dig deeper.

First, any high-fiber food (think apples, pears, high-fiber cereals, and legumes) helps trim fat off thighs and hips. Why? Dietary fiber whisks excess estrogen from the body, and estrogen is notorious for directing fat toward your thighs and hips. This is a true breakthrough, because many diets of late have talked about banishing belly fat to the point of overkill. A lot of women I know would gladly slim their butts and hips over their bellies if given the right info. Well, now we have the nutritional solution.

WE BROKE THROUGH!: Testimonials from Dieters Who Lost Pounds and Inches Through Contour Foods

Taylor: Today is my final day on Cycle 1. My stats: I have lost 14 pounds. Also, I am down an inch in my waist and chest. I am down an inch and a half in my hips. I feel great.

   Collette: I am on Day 16 with a loss of 11 pounds. Who would have guessed?

I have to say that this plan works, and I am looking forward to baking and enjoying one of Dr. Mike's Power Cookies!

Martin: I can't wait for Cycle 2. I have a couple of days left on Cycle 1, and I am down 11 pounds and 10 inches in total! It really works!!

Jake: I lost 9 pounds on Cycle 1. My clothes are definitely fitting better and some are loose. That means inches lost!

Scott: After I started Cycle 2, I had the eating plan memorized. I didn't need to open the book and just stuck to the approved food. I hit my goal weight after losing 25 pounds. I've dropped almost 10 more since then. I've basically stopped eating sugar and carbs. I have my evening wine, have beer and pizza on occasion, and I really don't even feel I'm sacrificing anything. This is a snap.

Margaret: Having good health makes all the difference and staying active is essential. I want to be around to see my great-grandkids and to enjoy life in my seventies and eighties. My primary reasons for trying to find something that might help me lose weight, and for trying everything for more than five years to do that. Nothing really worked (but my efforts may have kept me from gaining even more) . . . no real changes in my shape . . . until the 17 Day Diet!

Corey: I started approximately 14 weeks ago and am now down 35 pounds now! Only 10 to 15 pounds away from my goal. I have to say this has been one of the easiest plans I have followed. I just love it and can tell it is something I will be able to keep up with. I have lost so many inches, and since I don't exercise much, I think it's got to be Dr. Mike's Contour Foods.

Lynda: I am 20 years old, and I have just started the diet with my mom. I am 5'3" and weigh 178 pounds. My goal weight is 130. I started three weeks ago and already my pants and dresses are too loose. I need to go shopping for smaller sizes!

I am quite humbled by these wonderful stories. I am even more humbled by the fact that science continues to support these results. Here's a study from Loma Linda University that backs me up. Researchers compared two groups—vegetarian women and nonvegetarian women—to see how their bodies reacted to their diets. The vegetarian women's diets were much higher in fiber, as you might suspect, than the other group. And the vegetarians had thinner thighs and less estrogen circulating in their bodies, leading the researchers to suggest that there is an inverse relationship between fiber and thigh circumference. Put another way, increasing fiber in your diet may decrease your thighs! This study was published in the *American Journal of Clinical Nutrition.*

A similar study, published in the *European Journal of Clinical Nutrition*, found that women who ate a diet high in vegetables, including legumes, monounsaturated fats, and fruits (a diet similar to the one in *The 17 Day Diet Breakthrough Edition*) had thinner thighs and hips than women who ate a lot of red meat. So there is good proof that you can slenderize your thighs by what you eat. While we're on the subject of thighs, it's worth adding here is that the 17 Day Diet is low in sugar and unhealthy fats, two nasty nutrients that contribute to cellulite, that unattractive dimpling that forms on thighs and hips.

I definitely do not want to downplay the importance of slimming down your belly. Even more compelling research has been done on how you diet your way to a trimmer waistline. Researchers have discovered a virtual arsenal of foods that burn belly fat: monounsaturated fats, such as olive oil and canola oil; whole grains; yogurt and other calcium-rich foods. All of these Contour Foods are part of the 17 Day Diet, and I'll point them out to you as we go through each cycle of this diet together.

I hope you like fish, because there is plenty of it on The 17 Day Diet. What scientists have discovered about fish is the following breakthrough: The healthy fats in fish shrink fat cells! That bodes well for changing the shape of your body overall.

I will be listing all the Contour Foods on each cycle, so as you make food choices, you'll want to pay close attention to these lists. If you're concerned about your thighs, select those foods that slenderize your thighs; if you don't like the way your tummy pooches, pick those foods that fight belly fat. What you'll find out throughout this journey is that you'll shave off inches from your entire body and emerge shapelier than ever.

The foods you'll eat on this diet can transform your body in ways you never thought possible—better proportions, less body fat, greater muscle tone and development, and more. I suggest taking a series of before-and-after photos of yourself from different angles. That way you'll be able to visually confirm for yourself that Contour Foods, integrated into *The 17 Day Diet Breakthrough Edition*, are truly making a difference in bringing back the contours in your body.

My goal is to help you become the best you can be. The diet, the Contour Foods, the workout, and everything in this plan will help you reach the physical and health goals you have always desired.

So, use foods to enhance your body shape! Here are my prescriptions for doing so.

For a Flatter Belly

- Choose monounsaturated fats: nuts and seeds, avocados, olive oil, canola oil, and flaxseed oil. (Pay attention to the Cycles in which these fats are included.) This prescription is based on studies documenting that monounsaturated fatty acids actually can help reduce belly fat, including what medical experts call *visceral* fat, which is packed around your vital organs. Visceral fat has been linked to a variety of diseases, including diabetes, breast cancer, heart disease, and dementia. At the same time, avoid saturated fats such as butter, animal fat and cream, and hydrogenated (trans) fats. These fats will slow down your metabolism, which runs counter to how this diet works.

- Enjoy probiotic and calcium-rich proteins such as yogurt and other such recommended foods. These foods help you to lose weight and have been shown in research to shrink your tummy. One reason is that they are high in calcium, a mineral fat-burner. With calcium in short supply, the body makes a hormone called *calcitriol*. This hormone transmits a message to fat cells and tells them to hang on to fat, especially around the belly. Eat the calcium-rich Contour Foods and you reverse the process.

- Depending on the cycle you're in, choose whole grains as your starch choices for most meals. Researchers have found that whole grains help trim fat around the waistline. I am talking about oatmeal, brown rice, wild rice, barley, bulgur wheat, whole-wheat bread, and whole-wheat pasta. Scientists aren't sure why these foods work such magic, but think it has to do with the contrast to what most people eat: highly processed refined grains. These foods are dismantled more quickly into sugars. When sugars inundate the bloodstream, insulin levels shoot up to help get those sugars into cells, where they are often stored as fat.

For Thinner Thighs and Hips

The key is to increase the fiber in your diet. As I have mentioned, a high-fiber diet has been shown to reduce fat-forming estrogen in the body. Scientists are not sure, but they think that by reducing estrogen naturally, with fiber, less fat gets deposited on the lower body.

The amount of fiber required to help trim your thighs is at least 26 grams per day. It is generally recommended that adults get 25 to 35 grams of fiber a day anyway. Among the most fibrous foods are beans, peas, lentils; rice, oat, barley, corn, and wheat bran; pears, apples, oranges, berries; carrots, potatoes, squash; seeds; nuts; whole-grain breads and cereals; and green beans, broccoli, spinach, tomatoes. All these foods are included on various cycles of the diet.

My women patients are always asking me what they can do about *cellulite*, an accumulation of fat cells that are trapped in the protein (collagen and elastin) fibers of the skin. All I can say is that some experts believe that fatty foods and sugar foods contribute to cellulite, and eating more light protein, fruit, vegetables, and fiber, while cutting out fatty and sugary foods, may help reduce cellulite. Exercising with weights is effective too; it makes your body more cellulite resistant.

Never forget that you cannot change your shape without working out. Fortunately, I have devised a breakthrough exercise program that truly does achieve spot reduction. Hand in hand with eating Contour Foods, imagine what your body will look like when you get to your goal!

Review

- *The 17 Day Diet Breakthrough Edition* emphasizes Contour Foods to help you change your shape.
- Note the Contour Foods listed under each cycle and plan your meals using them.
- Add my breakthrough Spot Reduction Workout to the diet and you'll improve your shape even faster.

PART TWO

· ·

The Cycles of Fat-Burning

4

The Fasting Breakthrough

B efore I explain the four cycles of the 17 Day Diet, I want to introduce you to one of the major new breakthroughs on the diet: optional Transitional Day Fast. Yes, you read that correctly: fast. Admit it: Someone mentions fasting and you think of images of pious-looking folk sitting in contorted positions chanting *ommmmm*.

I understand your hesitation. I myself love to eat so much that I contemplate my next meal before finishing the last. Even so, I know people who periodically fast. They're in terrific shape, and I love their strength of purpose and tenacity. So I looked into this fasting thing. Buddha did it. So did Jesus, for 40 days. In fact, the Bible mentions fasting 74 times. Greek physicians like Socrates and Hippocrates fasted for therapy, and the Muslims observe Ramadan for spiritual cleansing. While many fast for spiritual reasons, it seems still others withhold food to cleanse their bodies of toxins and lose weight.

I dug into the scientific research about fasting, which has been studied at least as far back as the sixties by medical professionals and nutrition experts. Back then, it was studied mostly using lab rats wanting to drop a few sizes.

What I found from a purely medical perspective is that the benefits of fasting are multifold. Here is a rundown.

Cardiovascular diseases have also shown dramatic improvements with proper monitored fasting. Fasting has also helped high blood pressure patients normalize their blood pressure without the use of medications. Gastrointestinal troubles respond well to this conservative care, too.

Fasting programs have helped people with type 2 diabetes normalize and regulate their sugar levels without medication. (Caveat: if you have this disease, talk to your doctor about your desire to fast and how you will go about it.) How can fasting affect blood sugar so positively? For one thing, fasting for a day breaks up the body's constant exposure to food and glucose.

Other benefits

- Higher fat-burning through the activation of certain hormones involved in metabolism
- Sparing of lean muscle
- Lower blood pressure
- Healthier cholesterol level
- Reduced levels of chronic inflammation, which is involved in many diseases

Because *The 17 Day Diet Breakthrough Edition* is about even more rapid results, I created an optional Transitional Day Fast between cycles to give you a little more fat-burning oomph. Basically, it involves drinking three Fat-Burn Smoothies throughout the day: one at breakfast, one at lunch, and one at dinner.

I call these *Fat-Burn Smoothies* because they contain ingredients that have been proven to help get rid of body fat:

Whey Protein

If you want to talk about another breakthrough in nutrition, let me bend your ear about whey, a component of milk. Whey is one of the most exciting nutritional discoveries in the food world today. But centuries ago, no one knew that. Cheesemakers once tossed it as a worthless by-product. Whey, made of mostly water, was dumped in local creeks and streams. The problem was that whey had enough protein, lactose (milk sugar), and other solids to clog the waste stream. In the 1960s, the feds started charging local municipalities a ton of dough to clean it up. Back then, whey was nothing more than trash.

It was so costly to clean up that they had to figure out something better to do with it. Some of the first whey innovators were in the field of sports nutrition; they realized that whey was a high-quality protein. One of the first discoveries was that supplementing with whey could help a weight-training person rebuild muscle.

But how, exactly? Upon further examination, it turned out that whey is rich in certain amino acids that have remarkable effects on health and performance. Its balance of essential amino acids, including branched-chain amino acids, nearly matches that of our skeletal muscles. *Branched chain aminos* are used by muscles for energy; they're so named because the molecular structure resembles that of a branching tree.

One of the branched-chain aminos is leucine. Studies demonstrate that leucine plays a key role in building muscle and helping muscles recover after exercise. In addition, whey protein is a source of cysteine, an amino acid that helps preserve lean muscle, particularly during exercise.

The studies showcasing how whey maintains and builds lean muscle led researchers to look into whether the protein plays a part in weight control. They found that whey helps reduce hunger and increase feelings of fullness. That's one of the reasons you'll be including whey on your fast. I don't want you to get hungry!

I count whey among my Contour Foods. A study conducted by the Beltsville Human Nutrition Research Center, published in the *Journal of Nutrition* in 2011, discovered that whey is an effective fat burner, and it helps decrease your waistline. This study is just one of many showing that whey is effective for weight loss

Whey proteins have an unusually rich supply of an amino acid called *tryptophan*, which is involved in making serotonin, a feel-good chemical, in the brain. If you're low in tryptophan, you can start craving carbs, sleeping poorly, acting impulsively (like wolfing down that food you shouldn't be eating), and being in a bad mood. Whey protein goes a long way to prevent these ill effects, so I think it's a near-perfect food for dieters.

Whey is also considered an *immunonutrient*. When given to hospitalized patients, it prevents harmful inflammation, fights germ invasions, strengthens immunity, and prevents muscle and bone wasting, according to a 2012 study published in *Current Opinion in Clinical Nutrition and Metabolic Care*. One of the reasons that whey is an immune booster is that it contains *glutamine*, an amino acid that strengthens the immune system and keeps your gastrointestinal tract healthy to prevent infiltration by germs.

It seems that whey is just about the perfect protein for the body, making it extremely nutritionally valuable. For the transitional day, you'll need to purchase a can of 100 percent whey protein powder, in vanilla.

I Did It the 17 Day Way!   Jenna

My total weight loss so far is 12½ pounds, and I am just thrilled. The weight came off quickly in Cycle 1 and with the fasting option. I just checked my calendar and realized that I have only been on this diet for 3 weeks. So these results seem fantastic to me.

The last five years I have been struggling to not gain any more weight, and forgot about losing. This strategy just wasn't working, although I tried everything. The scale had become an enemy and now it is a weight loss tool, spurring me onward.

Seeing results from the diet has been the biggest boost to my morale, and a *big* payback for all those willpower moments when I have been strong and able to keep on the program.

If you're just beginning the diet, and, if you follow it closely, once you get to day 5 or 6, all of a sudden you are on a roll. At that point, my old carb cravings were gone and I was not hungry. I ate the fruit and probiotic snacks as instructed.

Yogurt was something totally new to me and so was drinking green tea during the day. Both are now parts of the diet I enjoy most. I'll be 64 next month, and I look and feel great.

Matcha Green Tea Powder

Matcha (rhymes with "got-cha") is a powdered green tea made by pulverizing tea leaves. So, when you sip matcha, you're ingesting the entire leaf instead of just steeping the leaves and removing them. A study in the 2003 *Journal of Chromatography* found that matcha contains up to 137 times more antioxidant power than other green teas; specifically, an abundance of a substance called *epigallocatechin gallate* (EGCG) that may help lower the risk of stroke, cardiovascular disease, and certain cancers. EGCGs are also excellent fat burners.

Matcha also contains more caffeine than other green teas, but you won't get the coffee jitters because the amino acid L-theanine found in matcha promotes a feeling of relaxed alertness.

Green teas are grown worldwide, but matcha is unique to Japan. It has a sweet taste and more flavorful and hardy when steeped in hot water to make tea. Here, you'll be using it in a smoothie, although it is very versatile and can be used in a variety of dishes, including ice cream.

The health benefits of matcha just stream on. In a study published in the *European Journal of Clinical Nutrition*, investigators discovered that people who consumed matcha daily for two months normalized their blood sugar and diastolic blood pressure. Matcha is sugar free and is an ideal drink for those who are watching their sugar levels, as well as for diabetics.

Ever had bad breath? Matcha to the rescue. Bad breath is quite common. Doctors refer to it as halitosis. Often you don't realize that your breath stinks, and it takes that quiet word from a co-worker or loved one to bring it to your attention. Even if you manage to impress someone on a first date with your personality, bad breath can make them rule out a second.

There are many reasons for bad breath, but the main one is not cleaning and flossing correctly. Food particles then get stuck in your gnashers, decompose, and start to smell. The first defense against bad breath is proper dental hygiene.

Scientists have studied other antihalitosis measures, such as mouthwash, gum, mints, toothpaste, parsley oil, and matcha to see how well they either deodorize the offending compounds or stop their formation. Mouthwash, gum, mints, and parsley oil scored about a B on both counts. Toothpaste banished bad breath, but didn't halt the stinky decomposition process. Only matcha excelled at both tasks. The secret: There's an antioxidant in matcha that cleans and deodorizes the mouth. So, end your meals with a cup of matcha green tea.

You can purchase matcha at most health food stores and Asian markets.

Probiotic Foods

I've talked throughout this book about the power of probiotics, such as yogurt, for fat loss, and they are a key breakthrough food on the 17 Day Diet. In a 2010 study, published in the *European Journal of Clinical Nutrition*, these so-called skinny bugs were found to reduce abdominal fat and body weight in overweight adults, making probiotics another effective Contour Food. There are many other studies that extol the weight-control virtues of probiotics. They appear to work by improving digestion and gobbling up calories that might otherwise be packed away as fat.

Some additional examples: People who had the highest intake of dairy foods, such as yogurt, lowered their risk of weight gain by 67 percent over a 10-year period, compared to those with the lowest intakes, according to research published in the *Journal of the American Medical Association*. Also, researchers at Harvard School of Public Health studied the relationship between specific foods and long-term weight gain in more than 120,000 men and women. After analyzing data from the 20 year follow-up, researchers concluded that yogurt was the food most associated with keeping weight off, even better than fruits, vegetables, and whole grains!

Eating yogurt is definitely a fat-burner. Researchers at the University of Tennessee randomly assigned 34 healthy obese participants 18 ounces of fat-free yogurt or one serving of dairy daily for 12 weeks. Both groups adhered to a similar calorie-reduced diet. At the end of the study, the yogurt group experienced an average weight loss of 14 pounds, compared to 11 pounds in the control group. Additionally, those who ate yogurt retained 31 percent more muscle mass and lost 81 percent more abdominal fat, which was reflected in a reduction of over 1.5 inches from the waist. By comparison, the control group lost 0.23 inches. This improvement is noteworthy, because visceral fat ups the risk for cardiovascular disease and type 2 diabetes.

The 17 Day Diet focuses on digestive health, so that you can metabolize calories more effectively. You can improve your digestive health by eating yogurt and other probiotic-containing foods. These foods can correct problems like constipation and diarrhea. Probiotics may also help you stimulate your immune system.

Also, some new evidence reveals that adding yogurt to your diet can protect against the development of several types of cancer, including those of the colon, bladder, and breast. In a study published in the *International Journal of Cancer*, a 35 percent reduction in colon cancer risk was found in those consuming the highest amount of yogurt compared to those with the lowest amount in more than 45,000 men and women over a 12-year period.

Other research has shown that yogurt offers powerful cardiovascular support. In a study involving more than 1,000 women aged 70 and older, those with the highest yogurt intake not only had higher HDL (good cholesterol) levels, but also significantly lower carotid artery thickness, a measurement of atherosclerosis, than those with the lowest intake.

I think you can see why I emphasize yogurt on this diet, and as a component of the Transitional Day Fast!

Fiber

Fiber is a recognized fat burner that works on multiple levels:

- Provides bulk and volume in your stomach, so it helps you feel full.
- Ushers excess calories from your body so that they won't be stored as fat.
- Stimulates the release of an appetite-suppressing hormone in your stomach called *cholecystokinin* (CCK). CCK talks to your appetite control center in the brain and tells it that your stomach is full.
- Controls your fat and sugar intake. Fiber-rich foods are low in fat-forming foods like bad fats and sugars. The more fiber you eat, the fewer fattening foods you eat.
- Helps regulate blood sugar. Fiber takes a long time to digest; this means fibrous foods release blood sugar more slowly. This action helps prevent swings in blood sugar, which can produce food cravings. If you have type 2 diabetes, you should definitely pay attention to increasing your daily fiber intake.
- Produces an automatic caloric deficit. Although we don't count calories on this diet, I'd like to tell you about an important calorie-related aspect of fiber. If you take in 35 grams of fiber a day (the amount recommended for weight loss), you'll automatically burn about 250 calories from the total calories you ate that day. The reason is that your body has to work hard to process fiber, and that work burns calories.
- May reduce the incidence of colon and breast cancers, and lower bad cholesterol levels.

It just makes good health sense to have plenty of fiber each day. Your digestive system needs it, and so does your waistline.

For the Transitional Day Fast, you'll want to have a powdered fiber supplement on hand. Some good ones are:

- Metamucil Clear & Natural. I like this because it's grit-free and perfect for smoothies. The serving size is 1 heaping teaspoon, which provides 5 grams of fiber.
- Benefiber. It contains 100 percent natural fiber, dissolves completely in noncarbonated beverages, and won't thicken the liquid. The serving size is 2 heaping teaspoons, which provides 3 grams of dietary fiber. This product is grit-free, too.
- Garden of Life Raw Fiber. This is a blend of various natural fibers derived from seeds and vegetables. The serving size is 1 scoop, which provides 9 grams of dietary fiber.

You can purchase any of these at pharmacies or health food stores.

Low-Sugar Ingredients

Most of the other ingredients—namely almond milk and berries—in these smoothies are all low in simple sugars and carbohydrates, giving them a low glycemic quality, which means it is digested fully by the body and used for energy. I really like almond milk for diets, by the way. It's lower in calories than skim milk. It's lactose-free, making it perfect for people with milk allergies. It has absolutely no cholesterol, and that's terrific for heart health. But, most of all, it tastes pretty darn good.

Here's how the Transitional Day Fast works.

Breakfast

. . . .

Smoothie #1

1 cup unsweetened almond milk

½ cup plain low-fat yogurt

1 scoop vanilla whey powder

1 serving powdered fiber

½ cup of crushed pineapple, canned in its own juice, but drained

½ frozen banana

Place the ingredients in a blender, and blend until smooth. Tip: Blend the mixture for several minutes. This adds air to the smoothie, which will make you feel fuller. Makes 1 serving.

Lunch

If you're doing your Transitional Day Fast on a weekday, and you work, make your smoothie ahead of time and freeze it in a Ziploc bag. Take it to work and place it in the fridge. When lunch rolls around, it will be ready to drink.

. . . .

Smoothie #2

1 cup plain low-fat yogurt

⅓ cup unsweetened almond milk

1 cup frozen strawberries

1 serving vanilla whey protein powder

1 serving powdered fiber

Truvia, to taste

Place the ingredients in a blender, and blend until smooth. Freeze. Makes 1 serving.

Dinner

• •

Smoothie #3

1 cup unsweetened almond milk   1 teaspoon matcha

½ cup frozen blueberries   ½ cup crushed ice

Large handful fresh spinach   Truvia, to taste

1 serving vanilla whey protein
    powder

Place the ingredients in a blender, and blend until smooth. Makes
1 serving.

Also, drink at least 8 cups of pure water, and enjoy 3 to 4 cups of green tea
throughout the day.

Remember that the Transitional Day Fast is optional. You don't have
to do it. You know what is right for your body. If you opt for it, you'll do
it after you complete Cycle 1, Cycle 2, and Cycle 3. There's another way
to use it: to get back on track. Let's say you blew the plan one day, or over
the weekend. Use the Transitional Day Fast as damage control. After a less-
than-stellar dieting weekend, follow the Transitional Day Fast on Monday.
Doing so will help cleanse your body of the junk you devoured over the
weekend and get you losing again. Then start your cycle on Tuesday.

The Transitional Day Fast is a tool, pure and simple. Try it, and see
how it works for you. It is a great weight-loss technique, and I think you'll
be pleased with your results.

Review

- The Transitional Day Fast is based on a liquid diet that contains
  proven fat-burning and appetite-suppressing ingredients.
- Use the fast for one day between cycles.
- If you've messed up on the diet and have gained weight, use the fast
  as a tool to drop weight quickly and get back on course.
- The fast is optional; however, using it will accelerate your results.

Cycle 1: Accelerate

N ow it's on to the cycles.

Dropping up to 10 or 12 pounds over the next 17 days is possible, and you can see impressive results quickly if you follow to the letter Cycle 1: Accelerate.

The trouble with most diets (besides being boring and making you crave fattening stuff that you can't eat) is that it's tricky to find one that helps you shed pounds quickly without compromising your nutrition—and ultimately your health and vitality. This cycle gets you on the road to lean quickly, plus it keeps you full, energetic, and motivated.

On this cycle you can eat unlimited protein—including meat, poultry, eggs, and fish, as well as many vegetables. You limit your carbohydrate intake by initially cutting out white bread, potatoes, pasta, rice, chocolate, biscuits, and sugary desserts and sweets. Fruit and fats are not banned, and that's good because they will add sweetness and flavor to your diet.

Cycle 1 is called Accelerate because its purpose is to trigger rapid weight loss in a healthy manner by mobilizing fat stores and flushing water and toxins from your system. The following are the things the Accelerate Cycle will be doing for you:

- Reducing carbohydrate intake slightly so that your body taps into its storage fat.

- Increasing protein intake so that your body goes into a fat-burning, body-contouring mode.

- Correcting improper digestion—a situation that can hold you back from fat burning.

- Providing rapid weight loss at the start, so that you have the incentive to keep going.

- Cutting out sugar, sweets, refined carbohydrates, and other substances that cause those dreaded highs and lows in blood sugar.

Once you've broken the cycle, your body will simply not crave them anymore. In this cycle, you're removing foods that don't work well for your body.

- Clearing your body of possible toxins. Pollutants in the body mess with both the thyroid gland, which helps regulate the body's metabolism, and the energy factories of cells (*mitochondria*), which convert nutrients into energy.

If you reach your goal the first 17 days, you can go right on to Cycle 4, maintenance. If you still have more weight to lose move on to Cycle 2: Activate, and enjoy even more foods for another 17 days. And then it's on to Cycle 3 for the next 17 days, a more liberal version of the first two cycles. And, if you're waiting for the day when I declare that cupcakes are part of your diet, that day arrives with Cycle 4, designed to keep your weight off with the reintroduction of your favorite foods into your life.

SCIENCE SAYS: Toxins and Metabolic Rate

Our livers act like Rodney Dangerfield. They probably go around saying: "I don't get no respect!" Day in and day out, we're exposed to toxins through drinking water, some foods, and other sources. The liver, the primary organ of metabolism, has to work overtime to detoxify these things out of the body. Also, these particular toxins are stored in your fat cells—so, as you start to shed pounds, they're released into your bloodstream.

According to the *American Journal of Physiology: Regulatory, Integrative and Comparative Physiology, 2001*, a team of Quebec researchers found that when toxins are released while overweight people are dieting, their *metabolic rate*— how fast the body burns calories—slows down considerably, even more than the slowdown often caused by dieting. Fortunately, many of the foods, particularly fruits and vegetables, on the 17 Day Diet are heroes at cleansing the body of toxins.

The Accelerate Cycle is the handiest diet tool you've got for getting—and keeping—your weight down. Look, if your diet goes AWOL for whatever reason—and you gain some weight back, you can always return to the Accelerate Cycle to get back on track. Do this and you'll keep getting closer to your ideal weight.

My Hunger/Fullness Meter

Your parents probably drilled into you that you were not allowed to leave the table unless you finished everything on your plate. That was good advice when portions were smaller, and everyone hated to waste food.

These days, most of us don't know when we're hungry and when we're full. We lose this ability by the time we reach kindergarten. And it's making us fat.

I have a solution: Dr. Mike's Hunger/Fullness Meter. The Fullness Meter is kind of like the pain scale doctors ask you about when you are in the hospital. Basically, you rate your hunger and fullness on a scale. This is not a new idea; there are lots of hunger scales out there. The problem with most is that they want you to rate your hunger on a scale of 0 to 10. That's too complicated. What is the difference between a 0 or a 1, or a 9 or a 10, anyway? You'd spend so much time trying to figure out your rating that you won't have time to eat.

I say it's simpler to use a hunger rating from 1 to 2; and a fullness rating from 3 to 4. Here's how mine works.

Hunger Meter

1. I'm a little hungry; my stomach feels as hollow as the promises of a politician. Eat now to prevent yourself from progressing to overeating later: Other leading indicators of mild hunger are slight stomach growling, mild headache, shakiness, and loss of concentration. If you aren't sure whether you're actually hungry, you're probably not. You may be confusing true hunger with boredom, fatigue, or thirst.

2. I'm so hungry I could eat the lining of an empty Spam can. My stomach is growling so loud it scared off a junkyard dog. I've got to get something to eat, and fast.

Don't let yourself get here. You'll be eating a package of Twinkies and guzzling Coke like crazy.

Fullness Meter

3. I'm starting to feel full. I will stop now so that I can save on my grocery bill.

You have entered that pleasant zone where you are no longer hungry but not quite full, either. Feel honorable about leaving a little room in your stomach. Try to keep yourself here at meals, never starving, never stuffed.

4. I'm so stuffed I'll have to waddle over to the couch to collapse.

You have eaten too much, even if it's all on your diet. Avoid this extreme; practice more restraint. Don't feel obligated to clean your plate, either. Stop eating as soon as your stomach feels full. Those extra bites of food that you're trying not to waste add unneeded calories.

As you go through your day and manage your mealtimes, ask yourself how hungry or full you are, based on my Hunger/Fullness Meter. Your goal is to listen to your body and let go of external cues, such as the clock, to tell you when, and how much, to eat.

General Guidelines for the Accelerate Cycle

- Follow the Accelerate Cycle for 17 days. If you reach your weight loss goal, move on to Cycle 4: Arrive. If you have more weight to lose, go on to the next Cycle: Activate.

- Your diet will consist of lean proteins, vegetables, low-sugar fruits, probiotic foods like yogurt, and good fats. Starchy foods such as potatoes, legumes, brown rice, corn, and oatmeal are not permitted on this cycle.

- Remove skin from chicken or turkey prior to cooking or purchase skinless poultry.

- About eggs: You may eat up to two eggs a day. But stick to no more than four yolks per week if your physician has diagnosed you with high cholesterol. Egg whites can be eaten without restriction.

- Enjoy fresh vegetables and fruits as much as possible. For convenience, frozen and canned items are fine, if chosen in moderation. They must be unsweetened, however.

- Do not eat any fruit after two in the afternoon. Fruit is a carb. The timing of carbohydrate intake is very important. I've found that carbs eaten early in the day supply the body with only enough fuel (in the form of glycogen stored in muscles) to energize the body the rest of the day. You'll find that this approach also improves your waistline. If you eat carbs in the evening, it's harder for the body to burn them off because you burn less energy in the evening. Those carbs might be stored as fat.

- Avoid alcohol and sugar in order to help your body eliminate toxins, improve digestion, and burn fat.
- Adopt the habit of drinking green tea. It contains some caffeine, but offers compounds that help burn fat.
- About probiotic foods: Research indicates that they boost the immune system and promote gut-cleansing bacteria. Probiotic foods are also thought to help the body burn fat. If you don't like yogurt, try the no-sugar-added fruit-flavored yogurt or cultured milk, such as low-fat acidophilus milk (it tastes just like regular low-fat milk). Otherwise, you can still get the friendly bacteria you need: Most health food stores sell capsules containing probiotics; follow the manufacturer's instructions for dosage.
- Eat slowly and only until full; do not overload your stomach.
- Drink eight 8-ounce glasses of pure water per day.
- Exercise at least 17 minutes per day. And please focus on my 17 Day Spot Reduction Workout.

PHILIP: I Broke Through!

I've always been overweight, but I'm 6'5", so I've always been able to hide it really well. I've tried every fad diet known to man, and failed miserably at them all! Six years ago, at the age of 22, I started to develop some serious back issues, which over time developed into 7 herniated and 2 compressed disks. At first I just dealt with it, but once my wife and I had kids, the pain really started to get to me, because I couldn't hold or play with them. In fact, the night we went to the hospital for her to give birth to our first son, my wife had to help me put my shoes on, because my back had gotten so bad.

Last year, I finally got tired of not being able to play with my kids, who are now 4 and 2. Doctors were just pumping me full of narcotics, so I decided it was time to try something myself. I had always known that if I dropped some weight it would likely help my back some, so it was time to do something about it. My mom and dad had done the 17 Day Diet, and were very successful. So, I gave it a shot. At this point, with my back condition, I had been in bed for 4 months, only able to get out to go to the bathroom. Within 2 days of doing the diet, my energy levels totally changed, and I was starting to feel different, and was able to get out of bed and play with my kids. I still remember the first day I went outside to play with them; they thought I was joking when I told them to put their shoes on! In the first week, I dropped 22 pounds! I was hooked!

When I started the diet, I weighed 330 pounds, and was wearing size 48 pants, and XXL shirts, I could only shop at Big and Tall stores, as other stores didn't carry my size. Today, I'm happy to say I weigh 250 pounds, and I'm wearing a size 38 pants and XL shirts. I still have about 25 pounds to hit my goal weight, but I'm getting there.

My back is still in pretty rough shape; sadly, no diet can fix herniated disks, but the 17 Day Diet has literally given me my life back. I went from spending my life, and more importantly, my kids' lives, in bed. I couldn't play with them, and that killed me. I hated saying to them, "Sorry boys, Daddy can't play today." But because of the 17 Day Diet, and the weight I've lost, and the energy I've gained, I'm outside playing with my boys daily, running around the yard, swimming in the pool, and just having fun! Thank you so much to Dr. Mike and the 17 Day Diet, you've helped me do something I never thought I could do!

Before   *After*

Take It Off: The Accelerate Cycle Food List

Lean Proteins

Here's where you'll be getting a lot of your fat-burning, body-contouring power. Eat all you want of the following proteins. They're freebies. The 17 Day Diet is high in protein because it stimulates the reduction of body fat.

Fish

Salmon, canned or fresh

Sole

Flounder

Catfish

Tilapia

Canned light tuna (in water)

Opt for wild-caught rather than farm-raised fish, which may have received doses of antibiotics. Avoid the bigger fish such as swordfish, shark, king mackerel, and albacore tuna: They are the most likely to carry metals like methylmercury, which is considered a toxin.

Poultry

Chicken breasts

Turkey breasts

Ground turkey, lean

Eggs (2 eggs = 1 serving)

Egg whites (4 egg whites = 1 serving)

Cleansing Vegetables

Eat all you want from the following list. They're freebies, too. I call these *cleansing vegetables* because they support detoxification in the intestines, blood and liver, and offer protective antioxidants. A few honorable mentions:

Cauliflower, cabbage, broccoli, and Brussels sprouts give you important *phytochemicals* (disease-fighting substances in plants), which help the liver detoxify various types of pollutants from the food supply, drugs, and the environment.

Asparagus, spinach, and okra are all super sources of *glutathione*, a healing nutrient that removes fat-soluble toxins from cells and helps fortify your immune system. (Cooked chicken is also high in glutathione.)

Spinach, broccoli, tomatoes, and Brussels sprouts are loaded with a powerful antioxidant called *alpha-lipoic acid*. It fights free radicals, and keeps your blood sugar in balance. People with diabetes should choose these veggies often.

Onions are packed with natural chemicals that protect against disease.

Greens have *diuretic properties* (which help you lose water weight), and their ability to stabilize blood sugar prevents binge eating.

Artichokes have a range of health-promoting benefits. This superfood is brimming with antioxidants, and two of the most potent are cynarin and silymarin. These two phytochemicals are thought to lower cholesterol, protect your liver from toxins, boost blood circulation, and aid digestion. The leaves and the yummy heart of the artichoke contain both of these phytochemicals.

Artichoke

Artichoke hearts

Asparagus

Bell peppers: green, orange, red, yellow

Broccoli

Brussels sprouts

Cabbage

Carrots

Cauliflower

Celery

Cucumbers

Eggplant

Garlic

Green beans

Green, leafy vegetables (including beet greens, turnip greens, collard greens)

Kale

Leeks

Lettuce, all varieties

Mushrooms

Okra

Onions

Parsley

Scallions

Spinach

Tomatoes

Watercress

LEAN 17: Maximize the Health Power of Fruits and Veggies

1. Look for fresh produce that is crisp and not wilted. Fresh = nutritious.

2. When buying fresh fruits, look for bruises. Bruising initiates a chemical reaction that saps the nutrient content.

3. When purchasing salad in a bag, look for a colorful medley of greens in the package. The more color, the more antioxidants and phytochemicals in the vegetables.

4. Always select the brightest, most colorful fruits and vegetables on the shelves. The brighter the color, the more vitamins and nutrients in the produce.

5. Go for darker shades of green when buying lettuce. Dark-leafed lettuce, like romaine, is richer in certain B vitamins than are lighter varieties of lettuce such as iceberg.

6. Buy certain vegetables such as onions and sweet peppers in all their various colors for a greater array of nutrients.

7. Purchase fresh fruits and vegetables in season when their flavor and nutrition are at peak levels.

8. Buy locally grown fruit and vegetables when you can. They tend to be more nutrient rich because they come right from the field. (A lot of nutrient loss occurs when produce is in transit for delivery to supermarkets.)

9. Berries are highly perishable. At the grocery store, look at the bottom of the container. Staining is a sign that the fruit has been bruised or is overripe. Nutrient loss has already set in, and the fruit will spoil rapidly.

10. Look for the brightest strawberries possible. A bright color signals exceptional nutrient quality. If berries show too much whiteness at their base, they're less nutritious.

11. Sniff berries to test for freshness. A pleasant aroma indicates good flavor, ripeness, and nutritional goodness.

12. Buy a variety of fruits and vegetables on the food lists. The greater the variety of foods you eat, the healthier your nutrition.

13. Eat fruits and vegetables raw whenever possible. Generally, raw produce is healthier. Exception to the raw rule: Cooked carrots and tomatoes yield more antioxidants.

14. Cook vegetables in the shortest time possible to preserve nutrients.

15. Steaming vegetables is a great way to keep nutrients from escaping.

16. Avoid thawing frozen fruits and vegetables prior to cooking. As foods thaw, microorganisms possibly present in food may begin to multiply, spoiling the food.

17. In most cases, avoid peeling. Nutrients and fiber are lost when produce is peeled.

Low-Sugar Fruit—2 Servings Daily

Low-sugar fruits are good sources of fiber that provide bulk and digest slowly, helping you feel full. They're also full of water, high in fiber, and superlow in calories, which makes them ideal for weight loss.

Apples

Berries, all types

Grapefruit

Oranges

Peaches

Pears

Plums

Prickly pear cactus

Prunes

Red grapes

Probiotic Foods—2 servings daily

Probiotics help balance your digestive system, resulting in an overall increase in the efficiency of digestion. Research shows that probiotics may also help fight obesity. If you've been under stress, taken antibiotics, or eaten a lot of foods packaged with preservatives, these things can kill off the beneficial bugs in your system—so eating more probiotic foods is a good idea.

There's no RDA for probiotics. To maintain health, a probiotic count of 5 to 10 billion is adequate. That may sound like a lot, but consider this: a 6 ounce serving of yogurt contains around 17 billion probiotics.

Yogurt, any type, including Greek-style, sugar-free fruit flavored; plain; and low-fat (6 oz. container = 1 serving)

Kefir: similar to a drinking-style yogurt; great for making smoothies (1 cup = 1 serving)

Low-fat acidophilus milk (1 cup = 1 serving)

Yakult (small 50-calorie bottle)

Breakstone LiveActive cottage cheese (½ cup = 1 serving)

Reduced salt miso dissolved in low-fat, low-sodium broth (1 tablespoon = 1 serving)

Tempeh, a fermented cake of pressed soybeans (4 oz. = 1 serving)

Sauerkraut (½ cup = 1 serving)

Kimchi (Korean fermented cabbage) (½ cup = 1 serving). Find it in Asian supermarkets or natural food stores, and enjoy a small amount as a side dish with meals.

MISTER M.D., CAN YOU PLEASE TELL ME

What If I Take a Medicine That Interacts with Grapefruit?

Grapefruit and grapefruit juice (which you do not drink on the 17 Day Diet) interacts with a few specific prescription drugs, and one is *statins*, taken to lower cholesterol. Grapefruit and grapefruit juice may prevent the liver from sufficiently breaking down the drug. That means there would a higher dose in the bloodstream. Most doctors know this.

This interaction was discovered in research studies back in the 1990s. A handful of these studies talked about the usual dose of grapefruit juice. But the usual dose was sometimes a whole quart a day! No one drinks that much grapefruit juice, even if grapefruit juice is your favorite food.

Personally, I like grapefruit. I eat it for its taste, vitamin C, and fiber. Plus, I like folding the grapefruit in half and squeezing the juice into a spoon.

What I tell my patients who take statins is that they may enjoy ½ grapefruit or 1 cup of grapefruit juice (no juice on the Accelerate Cycle of the 17 Day Diet, though) in the morning.

Second, I instruct them to always take their statins in the evening. These measures help minimize any grapefruit-drug interaction. And they still get to squeeze their grapefruit.

Before doing these things, you should make sure to consult with your physician.

Friendly Fats: 1 to 2 Tablespoons Daily

I don't purposely tell my patients to eat fats, unless it's the healthy kind, such as fish oil (from supplements), olive oil, or flaxseed oil. These fats have some great benefits: Studies suggest that they can help reduce the risk of heart disease, stroke, certain cancers, and diabetes; they promote joint health; and they help you to lose weight.

Olive oil

Flaxseed oil

Condiments

Condiments and seasonings are allowed in moderation: salsa; low-carb marinara sauce; lite soy sauce; low-carb ketchup; fat-free sour cream; low-fat, low-sodium broth; Truvia or Nectresse (non-caloric sweeteners made from natural ingredients); sugar-free jams and jellies; vegetable cooking spray; fat-free cheeses; fat-free salad dressing; salt; pepper; vinegar; mustard; herbs; and spices.

Contour Foods on Cycle 1	
The Foods	*How They Work*
Fish	Fish contains omega-3 fatty acids, which help shrink fat cells and assist in burning fat around the abdominal area.
Pears and apples	Both fruits are high in fiber, which helps whisk excess estrogen from the body. Estrogen helps lay down fat on a woman's lower body, namely her thighs and hips.
Olive oil	This friendly fat helps prevent fat from building up on the waistline.
Yogurt	Yogurt and the calcium it contains are known to prevent fat from congregating around your tummy.

Meal Planning Made Easy

It's easy to remember what to eat during this cycle:

- As much as you want of specific proteins and cleansing vegetables.
- Supplement these foods with 2 low-sugar fruits daily; 2 servings of probiotic foods such as yogurt, kefir, Yakult (small 50-calorie bottle), acidophilus milk, reduced salt miso dissolved in low-fat, low-sodium broth, sauerkraut (½ cup serving), and 1 to 2 tablespoons of friendly fat. It's that easy.

You do not have to count anything, except your 2 fruit daily servings, your 2 daily probiotic servings, and your fat serving.

Here is a typical day on the Accelerate Cycle.

Breakfast

- 2 eggs or 4 egg whites, prepared without oil, or 1 serving probiotic food such as yogurt
- 1 fruit serving
- 1 cup green tea

Lunch

- Liberal amounts of protein in the form of fish, poultry, or eggs plus unlimited amounts of cleansing vegetables, or 1 probiotic serving plus unlimited amounts of cleansing vegetables
- 1 cup green tea

Dinner

- Liberal amounts of protein in the form of fish or chicken
- Unlimited amounts of cleansing vegetables
- 1 cup green tea

Snacks

- 2nd fruit serving
- 2nd probiotic serving

Additional

- 1 serving (1 to 2 tablespoons of friendly fat to use on salads, vegetables, or for cooking)

MISTER M.D., CAN YOU PLEASE TELL ME

Can I Take a Probiotic Supplement Instead of Eating Probiotic Foods?

Yes. Probiotics come in supplement form that you can buy at your pharmacy or health food store. Look for a probiotic supplement that contains 10 to 20 billion colony-forming units (CFUs). These supplements usually need to be kept in the fridge. Read the label to learn how to store it.

17 Sample Menus

Here are examples of how you can create your daily menu during the Accelerate Cycle. You may follow these exactly or create your own menus based on the above guidelines. Some days include easy-to-make recipes. You'll find these in the appendix.

Wake-up Drink

Every morning, as soon as you rise, drink one 8-ounce cup of hot water. Squeeze a whole lemon into the cup; the lemon stimulates your digestive system. Your goal is to drink at least seven more glasses of water by the end of the day.

The speed at which you burn calories slows down if you're dehydrated. And if you're dehydrated, your body can't take up nutrients like it needs to. Negative waters, such as coffee or tea, do not count toward your total daily fluid intake.

Consult your physician regarding the amount of your daily water intake if you have been diagnosed with congestive heart failure. Water requirements vary.

Day 1

Breakfast

- 2 scrambled egg whites
- ½ grapefruit, or other fresh fruit
- 1 cup of green tea

Lunch

- Large green salad topped with tuna, drizzled with 1 tablespoon of olive or flaxseed oil and 2 tablespoons balsamic vinegar
- 1 cup green tea

Dinner

- Plenty of grilled chicken with liberal amounts of any vegetables from the list, steamed or raw
- 1 cup green tea

Snacks

- 6 ounces no-sugar-added plain yogurt mixed with 1 to 2 tablespoons sugar-free jam or other probiotic serving
- 1 serving fruit from the list

Day 2

Breakfast

- 6 ounces plain low-fat yogurt, mixed with 1 cup berries or other fruit (chopped) on the list. You may sweeten the mixture with 1 packet of Truvia or sugar-free fruit jam.
- 1 cup green tea

Lunch

- *Super Salad*
- 1 cup green tea

Dinner

- *Elegant Poached Salmon with Dill Sauce* with liberal amounts of any vegetables from the list, steamed or raw
- 1 cup green tea

Snacks

- 6 ounces sugar-free fruit-flavored yogurt or 1 cup plain low-fat yogurt, sweetened with Truvia or a tablespoon of sugar-free fruit jam
- 1 serving fruit

Day 3

Breakfast

- 2 hard-boiled or poached eggs
- ½ grapefruit or other fresh fruit in season
- 1 cup green tea

Lunch

- 1 large bowl *Chicken-Vegetable Soup*
- 1 cup green tea

Dinner

- Plenty of roasted turkey breast or turkey tenderloin, steamed carrots, and steamed asparagus
- 1 cup green tea

Snacks

- 6 ounces plain low-fat yogurt, sweetened with Truvia or a tablespoon of sugar-free fruit jam
- *Kefir Smoothie*

Day 4

Breakfast

- *Kefir Smoothie*
- 1 cup green tea

Lunch

- *Marinated Vegetable Salad* or *Super Salad*
- 6 ounces plain low-fat yogurt with a sliced fresh peach, or other fruit in season, for dessert
- 1 cup green tea

Dinner

- *Eggplant Parmesan*
- Alternative dinner: Any of the lean proteins with plenty of cooked cleansing vegetables from the list
- 1 cup green tea

Day 5

Breakfast

- 2 scrambled egg whites
- ½ grapefruit or other fresh fruit in season
- 1 cup green tea

Lunch

- Salad of baby spinach leaves, grape tomatoes, and crumbled low-fat feta or blue cheese, drizzled with 1 tablespoon olive or flaxseed oil and 2 tablespoons balsamic vinegar
- 1 cup green tea

Dinner

- Ground turkey patties, with *Crunchy Salad*
- 1 cup green tea

Snacks

- 1 cup fresh berries
- 6 ounces plain low-fat yogurt, sweetened with Truvia or a tablespoon of sugar-free fruit jam

Day 6

Breakfast

- 6 ounces plain low-fat yogurt, mixed with 1 cup berries or other fruit (chopped) on the list. You may sweeten with 1 packet of Truvia or a tablespoon of sugar-free fruit jam.
- 1 cup green tea

Lunch

- *Lettuce Wraps* or grilled chicken breast with tossed salad drizzled with 1 tablespoon olive or flaxseed oil and 2 tablespoons balsamic vinegar
- 1 cup green tea

Dinner

- *Sesame Fish*, or any grilled or baked fish
- Steamed cleansing vegetables
- 1 cup green tea

Snacks

- 2nd fruit serving of your choice
- 2nd probiotic serving of your choice

Day 7

Breakfast

- 2 scrambled eggs, 4 scrambled egg whites, or 1 scrambled egg plus 2 scrambled egg whites. Top with salsa, if desired.
- 1 apple or 1 cup fresh berries
- 1 cup green tea

Lunch

- *Taco Salad*
- 1 cup green tea

Dinner

- A stir-fry of vegetables (broccoli, onions, julienne carrots, red pepper, etc.), and chicken strips with 1 tablespoon of olive oil. Season with a little garlic, ginger, and light soy sauce.
- 1 cup green tea

Snacks

- 2nd fruit serving plus 1 probiotic serving of your choice
- 2nd probiotic serving of your choice

Day 8

Breakfast

- 6 ounces plain low-fat yogurt, mixed with 1 cup berries or other fruit (chopped) on the list. You may sweeten the mixture with 1 packet of Truvia or a tablespoon of sugar-free fruit jam.
- 1 cup green tea

Lunch

- Salmon salad: 2 cups salad vegetables (lettuce, tomatoes, onions, cucumbers, etc.), baked or canned salmon, drizzled with 1 tablespoon olive or flaxseed oil, mixed with 2 tablespoons balsamic vinegar and seasonings.
- 1 cup green tea

Dinner

- Turkey burgers (made with lean ground turkey)
- Steamed vegetables (choose from list of cleansing vegetables)
- Side salad drizzled with 1 tablespoon olive or flaxseed oil, mixed with 2 tablespoons balsamic vinegar and seasonings
- 1 cup green tea

Snacks

- 2nd fruit serving
- 2nd probiotic serving

Day 9

Breakfast

- *Greek Egg Scramble*
- 1 fresh orange
- 1 cup green tea

Lunch

- *Salade Nicoise*
- 1 cup green tea

Dinner

- Grilled chicken breast (marinate in fat-free Italian dressing, then broil or grill)
- Steamed vegetables (choose from list of cleansing vegetables)
- 1 cup green tea

Snacks

- *Kefir Smoothie*
- 2nd probiotic serving

Day 10

Breakfast

- ½ cup Breakstone LiveActive cottage cheese
- 1 medium pear, sliced
- 1 cup green tea

Lunch

- *Balsamic Artichoke* (use nonfat salad dressing as a dipping sauce)
- 1 medium apple
- 1 cup green tea

Dinner

- *Oven Barbecued Chicken Breast*
- *Southwest Slaw*
- 1 cup green tea

Snacks

- 2nd probiotic serving
- Raw, cut-up veggies

Day 11

Breakfast

- Yogurt Smoothie: ½ cup acidophilus milk, ½ carton no-sugar-added fruit-flavored yogurt, and 1 cup berries (mix in a blender)
- 1 cup green tea

Lunch

- *Super Salad*
- 1 cup green tea

Dinner

- *Turkey Chili*
- Side salad drizzled with 1 tablespoon olive or flaxseed oil, mixed with 2 tablespoons balsamic vinegar and seasonings
- 1 cup green tea

Snacks

- 2 probiotic servings

Day 12

Breakfast

- 2 hard-boiled or poached eggs
- ½ grapefruit or other fresh fruit in season
- 1 cup green tea

Lunch

- Baked or grilled chicken breast
- *Ful-licious Salad*
- 1 medium orange
- 1 cup green tea

Dinner

- Baked or grilled fish, any kind from the list
- *Oven Roasted Vegetables*
- 1 cup green tea

Snacks

- *Kefir Smoothie:* Mix 1 cup kefir with 1 cup frozen unsweetened berries, sugar-free fruit jam, and 1 tablespoon flaxseed oil. Blend until smooth.
- *Choco Mint Ice Cream*

Day 13

Breakfast

- *Kefir Smoothie*
- 1 cup green tea

Lunch

- Tuna tossed with 1 tablespoon olive oil and 1 tablespoon vinegar, served over a generous bed of lettuce
- 1 cup green tea

Dinner

- *Easy Gourmet Chicken*
- Tomato and onion salad, tossed with fat-free salad dressing
- 1 cup green tea

Snacks

- *Poached Pears and Oranges*
- 2nd probiotic serving

Day 14

Breakfast

- 2 scrambled eggs, 4 scrambled egg whites, or 1 scrambled egg plus 2 scrambled egg whites. Top with salsa, if desired.
- 1 apple or 1 cup fresh berries
- 1 cup green tea

Lunch

- 1 large bowl *Chicken-Vegetable Soup*
- 1 cup green tea

Dinner

- Plenty of grilled chicken or fish
- Generous portion of mixed steamed vegetables
- 1 cup green tea

Snacks

- 1 medium pear or other fruit in season
- 2nd probiotic serving of your choice

Day 15

Breakfast

- ½ cup Breakstone LiveActive cottage cheese
- 1 medium pear, sliced
- 1 cup green tea

Lunch

- *Eggplant Parmesan*
- 1 cup green tea

Dinner

- Plenty of broiled lean ground turkey
- *Marinated Vegetable Salad*
- 1 cup green tea

Snacks

- 2nd fruit serving of your choice
- 2nd probiotic serving of your choice

Day 16

Breakfast

- *Spanish Omelet*
- ½ grapefruit or 1 medium orange
- 1 cup green tea

Lunch

- *Spicy Yogurt Dip and Veggies*
- 1 cup green tea

Dinner

- Plenty of roasted turkey breast or turkey tenderloin, steamed carrots, and steamed asparagus
- 1 cup green tea

Snacks

- 1 piece fresh fruit
- 6 ounce plain low-fat yogurt, mixed with 1 cup berries or other fruit (chopped) on the list. You may sweeten the mixture with 1 packet of Truvia or a tablespoon of sugar-free fruit jam.

Day 17

Breakfast

- Smoothie: 1 cup acidophilus milk and 1 cup berries (mix in a blender)
- 1 cup green tea

Lunch

- *Super Salad*
- 1 cup green tea

Dinner

- Steamed flounder or sole with lemon pepper
- Steamed broccoli
- 1 cup green tea

Snacks

- 1 medium apple or other fruit in season
- 2nd probiotic serving of your choice

Accelerate Cycle Worksheet

It may help you to plan your meals using the following worksheet. Using the food lists, simply fill in what you will eat each day.

Breakfast

Protein or probiotic serving: _____

Fruit serving: _____

Lunch

Protein or probiotic serving: _____

Cleansing vegetables: _____

Dinner

Protein serving: _____

Cleansing vegetables: _____

Snacks

2nd fruit serving: _____

2nd probiotic serving: _____

Other

Friendly fat serving: _____

Your Optional Transitional Day Fast

Now that you've completed Cycle 1, you may want to opt for a Transitional Day Fast. Remember, it involves having three liquid meals on that day.

Breakfast

. . . .

Smoothie #1

1 cup unsweetened almond milk

½ cup plain low-fat yogurt

1 scoop vanilla whey powder

1 serving powdered fiber

½ cup crushed pineapple, canned in its own juice, drained

½ frozen banana

Place the ingredients in a blender, and blend until smooth. Tip: Blend the mixture for several minutes. This adds air to the smoothie, and the extra air will make you feel fuller. Makes 1 serving.

Lunch

If you're doing your Transitional Day Fast on a weekday, and you work, make your smoothie ahead of time and freeze it in a Ziploc bag. Take it to work and place it in a fridge. When lunch rolls around, it will be ready to drink.

. . . .

Smoothie #2

1 cup plain low-fat yogurt

⅓ cup unsweetened almond milk

1 cup frozen strawberries

1 serving vanilla whey protein powder

1 serving powdered fiber

Truvia, to taste

Place the ingredients in a blender, and blend until smooth. Freeze. Makes 1 serving.

Dinner

. . . .

Smoothie #3

1 cup unsweetened almond milk

½ cup frozen blueberries

Large handful fresh spinach

1 serving vanilla whey protein
  powder

1 teaspoon matcha

½ cup crushed ice

Truvia, to taste

Place the ingredients in a blender, and blend until smooth. Makes
1 serving.

Also, drink at least 8 cups of pure water, and enjoy 3 to 4 cups of green tea
throughout the day.

. . . .

As you go through Cycle 1, let me say that your eating habits may be a lot
closer to horrible than healthy right now. That means it's time to hand out
pink slips to doughnuts, pizzas, super burgers, shakes, and fries. Your stomach is about to welcome some healthier inhabitants, and I'm going to help
you understand what it's like to feel good, and understand the connection
between the choices you make and how you feel. For the first 17 days that
you follow this diet, you will experience an entirely new energy, and you
will see how quickly it can happen and how much better you can feel.

See you (hopefully less of you) in 17 days!

Review

- Cycle 1: Accelerate—jump-starts your weight loss.
- This Cycle reduces carb intake slightly and increases protein intake.
- This Cycle clears your body of sugars and toxins to pave the way for
  weight loss.
- Use my Hunger/Fullness Meter to help you eat just the right amount
  of food for your body.
- Use this Cycle as a tool to re-ignite weight loss if you ever have a slip
  and need to get back on track.
- Finish the Cycle off with a Transitional Day Fast, if you wish.

6

Cycle 2: Activate

I f you've been on other diets, you're all too aware of the usual outcome: You cut back on your food and you lose weight, at least initially. But then, losing pounds slows to a crawl, before lagging or sometimes stopping altogether. Your body's natural defense tendency to preserve itself and its fat, at all costs, kicks in. The Activate Cycle corrects this, resetting your metabolism, so that your body stays in a fat-burning mode.

This cycle is easy to follow, too: You alternate your Cycle 1: Accelerate days with Cycle 2: Activate days. In other words, you work this cycle by spending one day on the Activate diet and the next on the Accelerate diet, switching between the two, one day at a time, as you progress toward your goal weight over the next 17 days. Another way to look at it: On odd days you stick to the Activate Cycle; on even days, the Accelerate Cycle.

The approach of alternating Accelerate days with Activate days, plus using the Transitional Day Fast at the end of each cycle, is based on the scientifically validated mechanism of *alternate-day fasting* (although there is no fasting on this diet in the true sense of the word). In a nutshell, this means alternating low-calorie days with higher-calorie days in order to lose body fat. Scientists at the University of California have led the way in this cutting-edge research, with both human and rat studies. (How many of these furry creatures have lost weight in order to save humanity from obesity during the past 50 years is a mystery to me.)

Publishing much of their research in recent issues of the *American Journal of Clinical Nutrition*, these scientists have unearthed intriguing findings. Alternate-day fasting can:

- Trigger sustained weight loss (no frustrating plateaus). The weight that is lost is mostly fat.
- Activate the so-called skinny gene, which tells cells to burn—rather than hold on to—fat.
- Reduce the risk of heart disease by lowering levels of bad cholesterol and triglycerides, decreasing blood pressure and lowering heart rate.

- Alternating your food intake is a powerful concept in weight management.

Here's a look at what this will be doing for you:

- Stripping away body fat. Your carb intake is still relatively low on this cycle. When you cut carbs, your muscles use carbohydrates (muscle glycogen) to compensate for energy. In general, low glycogen levels mean that your fuel tanks are running on empty, so the body switches over to an alternate fuel source to burn: fat. And that means fat loss. Therefore, cutting carbs is a bona fide way to burn fat.

- Giving momentum to your metabolism. This potent diet strategy seems to keep the metabolism elevated. It keeps your body confused, as opposed to letting it get used to one particular way of eating day after day. Just as you need to alter your workouts to avoid plateaus, you mustn't let your body get too comfortable with the foods you eat. It's all about shocking the metabolism to keep it stoked.

- Taming your appetite. On the Activate Cycle, you get to eat some starchy carbs. But not just any carbs. You'll eat natural, slow-digesting carbs such as oatmeal, whole grains, brown rice, beans and legumes, and sweet potatoes—a whole slew of carbs. Slow carbs take longer to get into the bloodstream from the stomach, which helps you feel full.

- Preventing carb sensitivity. Carbs are beneficial in that they help set up the body hormonally for muscle toning if you exercise. They spark the release of insulin, which ushers protein and carbs into muscles for growth and repair. However, if you overeat carbs, they can be readily converted to body fat and stored. On the Activate Cycle, you're limited to no more than two servings of slow, natural carbs a day. This is the amount most people—especially women—are physiologically capable of tolerating in order to sustain fat metabolism.

Another major difference between the two cycles is that you get to enjoy a greater variety of lean proteins, including shellfish and beef.

MADALYN: I Broke Through!

I came home for Thanksgiving last November to see that my mother and sister-in-law had both lost 30 pounds in the previous month. After I asked them how they did it, they explained that they started the 17 Day Diet. My mother gave me a copy of her book to read while I was in town.

The next morning, I hauled myself to the scale in her bathroom. Before I knew it, tears were rolling down my cheeks. I weighed 215 pounds. I had never weighed so much in my life. I traveled almost every weekend for my job, and I do love a cocktail (or three) with my dinner, but I hadn't realized just how badly I had let myself go. It was that moment that I knew I had to change my life, and the 17 Day Diet was the key.

Instead of resolving to lose weight with the New Year, I promised myself that I would start the day after I got back home from Thanksgiving. The first few days were hard; I felt like giving up. I wanted to go drinking with my friends. But in those moments, I would either call my mother for support or eat more of the foods allowed on Cycle 1. Before I knew it, 17 days had passed. I had lost 15 pounds. That was the momentum I needed.

I posted my weight on my Facebook page weekly. The support network I created with my friends was one of the major factors keeping me going. I would travel to an event for my job, and people would be amazed to see me and the progress I was making. I was becoming an inspiration and everyone asked me how I did it. You better believe I told them about the 17 Day Diet!

At the beginning of the New Year, I weighed 195 pounds. I had already lost 20 pounds that I wouldn't have, had I waited to start with my New Year's Resolution. I kept on pushing through. By May, I had reached the lowest weight I had been since I first became overweight: about 160 pounds.

I sat on my couch and cried the second I stepped off my scale. But this time, I was crying tears of joy and pride. I had made it so far, and my hard work was paying off so well. Fast forward a couple of months: I had a really hectic work schedule that included being gone from home for every weekend in June. I began to make some poor choices and have now gained back a little bit of the weight I had lost. Today, I began Cycle 1 again, because I know that this program works. Because it's not a diet; it's a lifestyle change. It taught me to be more aware of what I put into my body and how to make better choices, so I don't step on a scale and see the number 215 again. I've joined a gym and I can walk up stairs without getting winded. My mother and sister-in-law have the same kind of success. My mother is 10 pounds away from her goal weight, and my sister-in-law is now training for a half marathon, all because we started turning our lives around with the help of the 17 Day Diet. It didn't just change my life. The 17 Day Diet saved my life.

Before   *After*

General Guidelines for the Activate Cycle

- Stay on the Activate Cycle for 17 days. The Activate Cycle consists of alternating between Activate days and Accelerate days.
- Remove skin from chicken or turkey before cooking, or purchase skinless poultry.
- Trim all visible fat from meat.
- About eggs: You may eat up to two eggs a day. Stick to no more than four yolks per week if your physician has diagnosed you with high cholesterol. Egg whites can be eaten without restriction.
- Keep gobbling those fresh fruits and vegetables before they become worthy of a science fair project in your fridge. For convenience, frozen and canned items are fine, if chosen in moderation. These products should be unsweetened.
- Continue to avoid alcohol and sugar in order to help your body eliminate toxins, improve digestion, and burn fat.
- Don't eat more than two servings daily from the natural starches list.
- Do not eat your fruit or natural starch serving past 2:00 p.m.

- Eat slowly and only until full; do not overload your stomach. Use my Hunger/Fullness Meter.
- Drink eight 8-ounce glasses of pure water per day.
- Exercise at least 17 minutes per day.

SCIENCE SAYS: Just a Single High-Fat Meal Does Heart Damage

Eating just one single high-fat meal makes your blood pressure go sky high, according to an April 2007 study by U.S. and Canadian researchers in the *Journal of Nutrition*. They fed 30 healthy people a single meal that was either very low-fat (1% of calories) or very high-fat (46% of calories). The high-fat meal was a McDonald's breakfast; the healthier, low-fat meal was cereal and nonfat yogurt. The people were then exposed to stressful situations, such as public speaking, doing arithmetic in their heads, and exposure to cold temperatures. Compared to the people given the low-fat meal, those who ate the high-fat meal had a greater hike in blood pressure and more stress on their blood vessels. These effects may cause harm to cardiovascular health. So much for the adage, "All things in moderation."

Take More Off: The Activate Cycle Food List

On the Activate Cycle, you'll be adding new foods to those you ate on the Accelerate Cycle. These additional foods are listed below.

Proteins

Add the following foods:

Shellfish

Clams

Crab

Mussels

Oysters

Scallops

Shrimp

Lean Cuts of Meat* (The leanest cuts are those from the part of the animal that gets the most exercise. Therefore, cuts from the round, chuck, shank, and flank are the best.)

Flank steak

Top sirloin steak

Top round

Eye of the round

Beef round tip

Beef top sirloin

Beef top loin

Lean ground beef

Pork tenderloin

Pork sirloin chops

Pork boneless loin roast

Pork top or center loin chops

Lamb shanks

Lamb sirloin roast

Veal cutlet

Natural Starches

Grains (1 serving = ½ cup)

Amaranth

Barley, pearled

Brown rice

Bulgur

Couscous

Cream of wheat

Grits

* Lean cuts tend to be a little tougher. You can tenderize lean cuts by marinating them in fat-free liquids like wine, fat-free salad dressings, or fat-free broth.

Long grain rice, such as Basmati

Millet

Oat bran

Old-fashioned oatmeal

Quinoa

Legumes (1 serving = ½ cup)

Black beans

Black-eyed peas

Butter beans

Garbanzo beans (chickpeas)

Great Northern beans

Kidney beans

Lentils

Lima beans, baby

Navy beans

Peas

Pinto beans

Soy beans

Split peas

Starchy Vegetables

Breadfruit (1 serving = 1 cup)

Corn (1 serving = ½ cup)

Potato (1 serving = 1 medium)

Pumpkin (1 serving = ½ cup)

Sweet potato (1 serving = 1 medium)

Taro (1 serving = ½ cup)

Winter squash (acorn, spaghetti, butternut, etc.) (1 serving = 1 cup)

Yam (1 serving = 1 medium)

Cleansing Vegetables

Same foods as Accelerate Cycle.

Low-Sugar Fruits

Same foods as Accelerate Cycle.

Probiotics

Same foods as Accelerate Cycle.

Friendly Fats

Same foods as Accelerate Cycle.

Condiments

Condiments and seasonings are allowed in moderation: salsa; low-carb marinara sauce; lite soy sauce; low-carb ketchup; fat-free sour cream; low-fat, low-sodium broth; Truvia or Nectresse (non-caloric sweeteners made from natural ingredients); sugar-free jams and jellies; vegetable cooking spray; fat-free cheeses; fat-free salad dressing; salt; pepper; vinegar; mustard; herbs; and spices.

Meal Planning Made Easy

On Activate days, you eat:

- Liberal amounts of protein and cleansing vegetables.
- Two daily servings of natural starches (carbohydrates).
- Two low-sugar fruit servings.
- Two servings of probiotic foods.
- One daily serving of friendly fat.

Here's a typical day on the Activate Cycle:

Breakfast

- ½ cup hot whole grain cereal or 2 eggs or 4 egg whites, prepared without oil; 1 *Dr. Mike's Power Cookie*; or one probiotic serving
- 1 fruit serving
- 1 cup green tea

Lunch

- Liberal amounts of protein in the form of fish, shellfish, meat, or chicken or eggs, or vegetables plus 1 probiotic serving
- 1 serving natural starch
- Unlimited amounts of cleansing vegetables
- 1 cup green tea

Dinner

- Liberal amounts of protein in the form of fish, shellfish, meat, or chicken or turkey
- Unlimited amounts of cleansing vegetables
- 1 cup green tea

Snacks

- 2nd fruit serving
- 2nd probiotic serving

Additional

- 1 friendly fat serving (1 to 2 tablespoons of olive oil or flaxseed oil to use on salads, vegetables, or for cooking)

Remember: Follow one day of the Activate Cycle with a menu from the Accelerate Cycle, and alternate accordingly for a total of 17 days.

Contour Foods on Cycle 2

In addition to the Contour Foods you ate on Cycle 1 (fish, pears, apples, olive oil, and yogurt), you'll now add the following foods to the mix.

The Foods	How They Work
Whole grains	Studies have shown that people who eat whole grains regularly have smaller waistlines than those who avoid these foods.
Legumes	Legumes are among the highest-fiber foods around. Remember, fiber reduces excess thigh-padding estrogen in the body.
Whey protein	This supplemental protein, which can be mixed into shakes, helps control abdominal fat, as well as fat all over the body.

17 Sample Menus

Here are examples of how to create your daily meals during the Activate Cycle. You may follow these exactly or create your own menus based on the above guidelines. Recipes are in the appendix.

Wake-up Drink

Every morning, as soon as you rise, drink one 8-ounce cup of hot water. Squeeze a lemon into the cup; the lemon stimulates your digestive system. Drink at least six to seven more glasses of water by the end of the day, more if you can. The rate at which you burn calories drops if you're dehydrated. And if you're dehydrated, your body doesn't absorb nutrients properly.

Day 1

Breakfast

- 1 *Dr. Mike's Power Cookie*
- 1 fresh peach, sliced
- 1 cup green tea

Lunch

- Chicken salad: baked or grilled chicken breast (diced), loose-leaf lettuce, 1 sliced tomato, assorted salad veggies, 2 tablespoons olive oil mixed with 4 tablespoons balsamic vinegar
- ½ cup brown rice
- 6 ounces no-sugar-added fruit-flavored yogurt

Dinner

- *Elegant Poached Salmon with Dill Sauce*
- *Oven Roasted Vegetables*

Snacks

- Protein Smoothie: 1 cup acidophilus milk or kefir blended with 1 cup frozen unsweetened berries

Day 2

- Accelerate Cycle menu

Day 3

Breakfast

- *Mexican Huevos*
- ½ grapefruit, or other fresh fruit of your choice
- 1 cup green tea

Lunch

- 1 large bowl of *Chicken-Vegetable Soup* or grilled chicken breast and plenty of steamed veggies
- 1 medium baked potato with 1 tablespoon fat-free sour cream (A medium potato fits in the palm of your hand.)
- 6 ounces no-sugar-added fruit-flavored yogurt
- 1 cup green tea

Dinner

- *Catalina Grilled Steak*
- Tossed salad with 1 tablespoon olive oil and 2 tablespoons balsamic vinegar
- 1 cup green tea

Snacks

- 1 cup fresh raspberries (or other in-season fruit) with 1 cup no-sugar-added fruit-flavored yogurt
- Mediterranean spread: ½ cup garbanzo beans (pureed and mixed with 1 tablespoon olive oil) served on cucumber slices

Day 4

- Accelerate Cycle menu

Day 5

Breakfast

- ½ cup oatmeal or grits, cooked
- 4 egg whites, scrambled
- 1 fresh peach, sliced
- 1 cup green tea

Lunch

- *Mexican-Style Shrimp*
- ½ cup brown rice
- 1 cup green tea

Dinner

- *Drunken Pork Chops*
- *Stewed Zucchini*
- 1 cup green tea

Snacks

- 1 cup blueberries with 6 ounces no-sugar-added fruit-flavored yogurt
- 6 ounces sugar-free fruit-flavored yogurt or 1 cup kefir

Day 6

- Accelerate Cycle menu

Day 7

Breakfast

- 2 eggs, scrambled without oil
- 1 medium potato, peeled, diced, and browned over medium heat in a small frying pan that has been coated with vegetable cooking spray
- 1 orange or other fresh fruit in season
- 1 cup green tea

Lunch

- *Black Bean Chili*
- *Cactus Salad*
- 1 cup green tea

Dinner

- *Old-Fashioned Beef Stew*
- 1 cup green tea

Snacks

- *Kefir Smoothie*
- 6 ounces no-sugar-added fruit-flavored yogurt

Day 8

- Accelerate Cycle menu

Day 9

Breakfast

- ½ cup Breakstone LiveActive cottage cheese
- 1 medium pear, sliced
- 1 cup green tea

Lunch

- Grilled chicken breast
- ½ cup *Picnic Beans* or ½ cup pinto beans
- ½ cup cooked corn
- 1 cup green tea

Dinner

- Grilled salmon
- Steamed broccoli
- Sliced fresh tomato drizzled with 1 tablespoon of olive or flaxseed oil mixed with vinegar and seasonings
- 1 cup green tea

Snacks

- 1 medium apple
- 6 ounces no-sugar-added fruit-flavored yogurt

Day 10

- Accelerate Cycle menu

Day 11

Breakfast

- *Kefir Smoothie* (blended with 1 cup berries)
- 1 cup green tea

Lunch

- Plenty of broiled hamburger
- *Guiltless Potato Salad*
- ½ cup peas

Dinner

- Plenty of roasted turkey breast
- *Asparagus Tarragon Salad*
- Large tossed salad with 1 tablespoon olive oil mixed with 2 tablespoons vinegar and seasoning

Snacks

- 1 medium orange
- 6 ounces no-sugar-added fruit-flavored yogurt

Day 12

- Accelerate Cycle menu

Day 13

Breakfast

- 1 *Harvest French Toast*
- 1 medium peach, sliced
- 1 cup green tea

Lunch

- *Low-Carb Primavera Delight*
- 1 cup green tea

Dinner

- *Apricot-Glazed Lamb Chops*
- Large tossed salad with 1 tablespoon olive oil mixed with 2 tablespoons vinegar and seasoning
- 1 cup green tea

Snacks

- Yogurt Shake (blended with fruit)
- 2nd probiotic serving of your choice

Day 14

- Accelerate Cycle menu

Day 15

Breakfast

- 1 cup *Lean Granola* mixed with 6 ounces no-sugar-added fruit-flavored yogurt (*Note:* 1 cup *Lean Granola* gives you your 2 servings of natural starch for the day.)
- 1 cup green tea

Lunch

- Fruit salad: ½ cup LiveActive Breakstone cottage cheese with diced fruit (½ cup diced strawberries and ½ cup diced peach) served on a generous bed of lettuce
- 1 cup green tea

Dinner

- *Chicken with Orange Sauce*
- Large tossed salad with 1 tablespoon olive oil mixed with 2 tablespoons vinegar and seasoning
- *Chocolate Candies* for dessert
- 1 cup green tea

Snacks

- 1 medium apple or pear
- 2nd probiotic serving of your choice

Day 16

- Accelerate Cycle menu

Day 17

Breakfast

- 2 cooked eggs (prepared without oil)
- 1 cup fresh berries
- 1 cup green tea

Lunch

- Grilled chicken breast
- 1 bowl *Pumpkin Soup*
- ½ cup cooked corn
- 1 cup green tea

(Note: The servings of sweet potato and/or squash plus corn give you your 2 servings of natural starch for the day.)

Dinner

- *Garlic Shrimp*
- Steamed green beans
- Large tossed salad with 1 tablespoon olive oil mixed with 2 tablespoons vinegar and seasoning
- 1 cup green tea

Snacks

- 1 medium orange or nectarine
- *Choco Mint Ice Cream*

LEAN 17: Lost in Spice—17 Ways to Make Veggies and Other Foods Taste Great

When you're on a diet, you've got to be creative. Here are some suggestions to get the most flavor from your food, without using added fat or sugar.

1. **Basil.** Basil adds loads of flavor to tomato-based dishes. It's also great with poultry.

2. **Broth.** Use low-sodium, low-fat chicken and beef broth to sauté meats and cook flavorful rice without adding oil.

3. **Cayenne pepper.** Just a pinch livens up chili, spaghetti squash, and salad dressings. Consuming cayenne may help suppress your appetite. When a group of men and women took 900 milligrams of cayenne pepper half an hour before meals, they felt fuller and reduced their calorie and fat intake, according to a study in the June 2005 issue of *International Journal of Obesity*.

4. **Chives.** Add 1 part chopped chives to 3 parts spinach and boil or steam for 3 minutes.

5. **Cinnamon.** Sprinkle this spice in oatmeal, hot cereals, or coffee. A 2003 study published in *Diabetes Care* reported that as little as one gram of cinnamon reduced blood glucose and cholesterol levels in type 2 diabetics.

6. **Dill.** Known mostly as a pickling herb, dill is delicious on fish, carrots, and salads. For an easy dip, mix it into plain yogurt and serve with cucumber slices.

7. **Garlic.** Stir it into mashed potatoes or salad dressing.

8. **Horseradish.** Ditch the gravy and go for horseradish to enliven meat. Or puree it with Breakstone LiveActive cottage cheese, along with some garlic and pepper, for a healthy vegetable dip or potato topping.

9. **Italian seasonings** (generally a combination of oregano, rosemary, savory, marjoram, basil, and thyme). Sprinkle it on chicken, spaghetti squash, tomatoes, and other vegetables.

10. **Lemon.** Squeeze fresh juice on salads, vegetables, and fish. Grate to remove the zest (flavorful outer rind), which gives a tang to poultry, vegetables, and salads.

11. **Mint.** You can't beat fresh mint from your garden, but dried mint is tasty, too. Good in tea, with fruit, and in plain yogurt.

12. **Mustard.** Dijon mustard adds zip to many dishes, from turkey burgers to roasted potatoes.

13. **Rosemary.** The fragrant, needlelike leaves of this woody herb are especially good with lamb and seafood, and in any dish with beans, tomatoes, onions, potatoes, or cauliflower.

14. **Sage.** This Mediterranean herb is especially good in tomato-based dishes, beans, tuna, chicken, or turkey.

15. **Tarragon.** This wonderful seasoning makes salads and chicken taste delicious. For your salad dressings, try tarragon vinegar mixed with olive oil or flaxseed oil.

16. **Thyme.** A member of the mint family, thyme is great on carrots, cauliflower, Brussels sprouts, and beef.

17. **Vinegar.** Try cider vinegar on cooked spinach, herbed or raspberry vinegar on salad greens, rice vinegar on chicken salad, and malt vinegar on broiled fish.

Activate Cycle Worksheet

It may help you to plan your meals using the following worksheet. Using the food lists, simply fill in what you will eat each day.

Activate Day

Breakfast

Protein or probiotic serving: _____

Natural starch serving: _____

Fruit serving: _____

Lunch

Protein or probiotic serving: _____

Natural starch serving: _____

Cleansing vegetables: _____

Dinner

Protein serving: _____

Cleansing vegetables: _____

Snacks

2nd fruit serving: _____

2nd probiotic serving: _____

Other

Friendly fat serving: _____

Accelerate Days

Breakfast

Protein or probiotic serving: _____

Fruit serving: _____

Lunch

Protein or probiotic serving: _____

Cleansing vegetables: _____

Dinner

Protein serving: _____

Cleansing vegetables: _____

Snacks

2nd fruit serving: _____

2nd probiotic serving: _____

Other

Friendly fat serving: _____

Your Optional Transitional Day Fast

Now that you've completed Cycle 2, you may want to opt for a Transitional Day Fast. Remember, it involves having three liquid meals on that day.

Breakfast

. . . .

Smoothie #1

1 cup unsweetened almond milk

½ cup plain low-fat yogurt

1 scoop vanilla whey powder

1 serving powdered fiber

½ cup crushed pineapple, canned in its own juice, drained

½ frozen banana

Place the ingredients in a blender, and blend until smooth. Tip: Blend the mixture for several minutes. This adds air to the smoothie, which will make you feel fuller. Makes 1 serving.

Lunch

If you're doing your Transitional Day Fast on a weekday, and you work, make your smoothie ahead of time and freeze it in a Ziploc bag. Take it to work and place it in a fridge. When lunch rolls around, it will be ready to drink.

. . . .

Smoothie #2

1 cup plain low-fat yogurt

⅓ cup unsweetened almond milk

1 cup frozen strawberries

1 serving vanilla whey protein powder

1 serving powdered fiber

Truvia, to taste

Place the ingredients in a blender, and blend until smooth. Freeze. Makes 1 serving.

Dinner

. . . .

Smoothie #3

1 cup unsweetened almond milk

½ cup frozen blueberries

Large handful fresh spinach

1 serving vanilla whey protein
    powder

1 teaspoon matcha

½ cup crushed ice

Truvia, to taste

Place the ingredients in a blender, and blend until smooth. Makes
1 serving.

Also, drink at least 8 cups of pure water, and enjoy 3 to 4 cups of green tea
throughout the day.

Review

- Cycle 2: Activate—is based on "alternate day fasting," in which you alternate lower-calorie days with slightly higher-calorie days. Here you alternate Activate days with Accelerate days.
- Alternating your diet days charges up your metabolism and helps prevent dreaded weight-loss plateaus.
- Additional foods such as natural carbs are re-introduced to your diet on this Cycle.
- You may want to opt for a Transitional Day Fast at the end of this cycle.

By the time you finish the Activate Cycle, provided you've done it without cheating, you'll have enough of a weight loss that your clothes are starting to get too baggy and loose for you. Don't lose focus now, because you're doing great.

Cycle 3: Achieve

You have been on the 17 Day Diet for 34 days. Yes, I'm counting. We should be seeing less of you, since French fries and candy bars are no longer homesteading on your hips. You're looking great, fitting beautifully into clothes, and (I hope) are pleased with your progress.

Now is the time to start adding new food choices, including items like pasta. Pasta is not the archenemy of the human body, by the way; portions the size of national monuments are. Every food group is represented on Cycle 3, and there's still an emphasis on nonstarchy vegetables and lean protein. Now, you can enjoy some alcohol, unless you're going to drive, you're under 21, you're pregnant, defusing a bomb, or working in a nuclear power plant.

On this cycle, you'll eat moderately, and continue to do some form of exercise that works your cardiovascular system, only I want you to step up the duration of your workouts.

There are fewer food rules on this cycle. But, yes, food eaten over the sink or stove, or otherwise while you're standing up, still counts in your daily intake.

I call this Cycle Achieve because one of its chief purposes is to help you achieve good lifetime eating habits, such as portion control, regular mealtimes, and the inclusion of healthy foods.

Some of you may have already reached your goal weight, particularly if you had just 10 or 15 pounds to take off. Congratulations. You may collect a Get-Out-of-the-Achieve-Cycle-Free Card and go right to Cycle 4.

CHECK-UP: Your Progress

☐ I have lost a pleasing number of pounds.

☐ My clothes fit better.

☐ I have dropped a dress or pants size.

☐ I have more energy.

☐ People have noticed my weight loss and complimented me.

☐ I feel more motivated to treat my body with respect.

☐ I feel less hungry.

☐ I am sleeping better.

☐ My skin looks better.

☐ My elimination has improved.

☐ My stomach is flatter.

☐ I feel lighter.

☐ I have fewer cravings.

☐ My mood is better.

For the rest of you, before we get started on Achieve Cycle 3, let's talk about what positive changes you've begun to enjoy. Look at my checkup on this page. Mark any changes that apply. Make a copy of the checklist and stick it on your fridge so that the next time you feel like nosing around in the freezer for that 20-inch pizza that you forgot to throw out, the list will stop you in your tracks.

The Speed of Weight Loss on Cycle 3

So far, you have been dropping weight at the speed of light, or just about. On Cycle 3, expect your weight loss to slow down a bit. I tell you this so that when you get on the scale, you won't be disappointed, blow your diet big time, and vow to not start up again until next January.

The goal of this cycle is to establish healthy eating habits and produce steady, manageable weight loss. Just relax and enjoy the addition of whole grain breads and pasta, additional fruits and vegetables, fats and snacks, and alcohol in moderation (one alcoholic drink a day).

Okay, now that I've told you your weight loss may slow down a bit over the next 17 days, let me tell you how to speed it up in Cycle 3. You can do this in these ways:

• Ramp up your aerobic exercise. Aerobic exercise, such as walking, jogging, biking, or classes, is the best way to burn fat and speed up weight loss. So, if you've been doing it at least 17 minutes a day, it's time to add even more minutes. Aim to do 45 to 60 minutes of aerobic exercise most days of the week.

- Include the 17 Day Spot Reduction Workout in your routine.
- Start my supplement program, outlined in Chapter 16.
- Consider doing my Transitional Day Fast every 7 days.
- Continue not to eat carbs after 2:00 p.m. During Cycles 1 and 2, I recommend not eating carbs after 2:00 p.m. If you did a good job of replenishing your muscle and liver glycogen throughout the day, which is what carbs do, then any excess carbs in the later afternoon and at night, a time when you're typically least active, will be readily converted to fat. On Cycle 3, you're allowed to have carbs at dinner. However, if you want to spur weight loss, continue avoiding carbs after 2:00 p.m.
- Pass on the alcohol. I know I just gave you the thumbs-up for alcohol on Cycle 3, but please know that alcohol can throw a complete monkey wrench into weight loss. Alcohol strains your liver, which responds by slowing down on functions like fat burning. Alcohol is also dehydrating and will cause water-weight pounds to register on the scale. If you want bigger losses during this cycle, pass up the alcohol option.

GAYLA: I Broke Through!

I was diagnosed with high blood pressure and placed on medication for two years prior to discovering the 17 Day Diet. I saw Dr. Mike on *The Doctors* and thought it might be something I could try. I was skeptical, of course, so I got the book from the library. I have been on all sorts of diets, have lost weight, and gained it back and then some. At my age (53) I thought it would be difficult to lose weight. Or so I thought.

A week after I had the book, I told a friend that I was thinking of starting a diet, and she emphatically said are you going to start? So, I felt I had to start immediately (the next day). In the first 17 days, I lost 18 pounds and was taken off of my blood pressure meds!

I persevered and continued for more than 6 months, and lost over 70 pounds. My cholesterol has dropped 30 points and is quite normal. My triglycerides cut almost in half, from 130 to 72. My blood sugar dropped as well, to 70. My doctor says I have been doing quite well by these numbers. I gained energy and have a better outlook. I am in much better shape than before. I have shared this with many people. I was once in a dressing room at a store, and my friend called me the incredible shrinking woman. A lady who was there wanted to know why she called me that. I explained the diet, and results, and gave her the name of the book. She was so happy; she said she thought her only chance was bariatric surgery. She had new hope after I spoke with her. Thanks, Dr. Mike, for putting together this diet. It is a life-changing thing for me. I learned many new things about healthful eating. And, I still expect to lose more weight. I am well on my way!

Before   *After*

Achieve Cycle Guidelines

- Stay on the Achieve Cycle for 17 days.
- Because you'll be eating more food, it's time to control your protein portions. Rather than eat protein liberally as in the two previous cycles, keep your portions of fish, poultry, and meat smaller—about the size of an average kitchen sponge. In fact, you can use that sponge to sop up any remnants of fat that might have dripped off the protein.

- Remove skin from chicken and turkey prior to cooking or purchase skinless poultry.

- Trim all visible fat from meat.

- You may eat up to two eggs per day; stick to no more than four yolks per week if your physician has diagnosed you with high cholesterol. Egg whites can be eaten without restriction.

- Enjoy fresh vegetables and fruits as much as possible. For convenience, frozen and canned items are fine, if used in moderation. Canned and frozen fruits should be unsweetened.

- You may have one alcoholic drink daily: 5 ounces wine, 12 ounces beer, or 1½ oz. hard liquor, if you wish. Attention, everyone reading this: Notice I said, "one." If you go to a party, have one drink, and spend the rest of the night drinking nonalcoholic, calorie-free drinks such as flavored seltzer. (This will help you avoid embarrassing work-party karaoke moments.) Please remember that alcohol has a dehydrating effect and can interfere with fat burning and weight loss. One drink per day, however, has a positive effect on cholesterol levels. Accumulating evidence suggests that moderate drinking may lower the risk of heart attack.

- Don't eat more than two servings daily from the natural starches list.

- Don't worry about eating all the food you're allowed each day. If you forget your second dairy or carb serving, or are too full to eat it, that's okay.

- Eat slowly and only until full; do not overload your stomach. Use my Hunger/Fullness meter as a gauge to keep you from stuffing yourself.

- Begin to increase your weekly aerobic exercise. Exercise at least 150 to 300 minutes per week, depending on your physical condition (five 30 minute sessions or five 60 minute sessions).

Achieve Cycle Expanded Food List

Where indicated, add foods to your diet, in addition to those you ate during the first 2 cycles.

Proteins

Fish and Shellfish (from Accelerate and Activate lists)

Lean Meats (from Accelerate and Activate lists)

Poultry (from Accelerate and Activate lists, including eggs and
   egg whites)

Additional poultry:

   Cornish hen

   Quail

   Pheasant

   Reduced-fat turkey bacon or turkey sausage or turkey lunch meat

Additional lean meats:

   Canadian bacon

SCIENCE SAYS: If You Have to Drink Alcohol on Your Diet, Drink Red Wine

Okay, here we are back on the alcohol issue. There is some intriguing research I want to share with you about one of my favorite food groups, red wine. I mentioned earlier that red wine contains a heart-protective compound called *resveratrol*, which does everything but fly to the moon. Apparently, resveratrol can also reduce the number of fat cells in a person's body, and scientists think it may one day be used to prevent obesity. Several years ago, researchers at the University of Ulm in Germany examined some human fat cell precursors, called *preadipocytes*. In the body, these are baby cells that develop into mature fat cells. They exposed the baby cells to resveratrol and found that the substance kept the pre-fat cells from multiplying and prevented them from converting into mature fat cells. Also, resveratrol impeded fat storage.

This makes sense, when you think about French women. French women are the skinniest in all of Europe, even though they eat a high-fat diet and drink lots of wine. Scientists think the resveratrol in red wine is a fat burner, according to the 2010 *American Journal of Clinical Nutrition*, and why the French can eat gobs of fat and still stay thin.

Natural Starches

Breads (1 slice = 1 serving)

Cracked wheat

Fiber-enriched bread

Gluten-free bread

Multigrain bread

Oat bran bread

Sugar-free bread

Pumpernickel

Rye bread

Whole-grain bagel (½ = 1 serving)

Whole-wheat pita, 1 pocket

Whole-wheat tortilla, 10"

High Fiber Cereals (1 cup = 1 serving, unless where indicated)

All-Bran

All-Bran Extra

All-Bran Bran Buds

Fiber One

Gluten-free cold cereals

Low-sugar granola (½ cup = 1 serving)

Pasta (½ cup = 1 serving)

Whole-wheat pasta

Gluten-free pasta

Vegetable-based pasta

High-fiber pasta

Udon noodles

Miracle noodles

Vegetables—Unlimited

All cleansing vegetables

Alfalfa

Broccoli sprouts

Chilies

Cilantro

Fennel

Grape leaves

Jicama

Kelp and other edible seaweeds

Kohlrabi

Nopales (edible cactus)

Pea pods

Radishes

Rhubarb

Rutabaga

Summer squash

Swiss chard

Yellow wax beans

Zucchini

Virtually any vegetable

Fruits—2 servings daily*

Apricots

Bananas

Cherries

Currants

Figs

Guava

* Serving = 1 piece fresh or 1 cup chopped fresh fruit.

Kiwi

Kumquats

Mango

Papaya

Pineapple

Pomegranate

Tangelo

Tangerine

Virtually any fresh fruit

If you are watching your sugar intake, stick to lower-sugar fruits. These include apples, berries (all varieties), cherries, grapefruit, orange, peach, pear, and plums.

Probiotics, Dairy, and Dairy Substitutes: 1 to 2 servings daily

Some people don't like dairy foods, or can't digest them properly. If you're one of them, try dairy substitutes, such as sugar-free rice, almond, or soy milk (1 cup = 1 serving). Try to eat at least one serving daily from this list while on the Achieve Cycle.

Probiotic Foods from Accelerate and Activate Cycles

Cheeses (Brie, Camembert, Fontina, low-fat Cheddar, Edam, feta, goat, Limburger, and part-skim mozzarella) (2 ounces = 1 serving)

Low-fat cottage cheese (½ cup = 1 serving)

Low-fat milk, including skim (1 cup = 1 serving)

Low-fat ricotta cheese (½ cup = 1 serving)

Friendly Fats—1 to 2 tablespoons daily, unless indicated elsewhere

Avocado (¼ fruit = 1 serving)

Canola oil (1 tablespoon = 1 serving)

Walnut oil (1 tablespoon = 1 serving)

Light mayonnaise (2 tablespoons = 1 serving)

Mayonnaise (1 tablespoon = 1 serving)

Nuts or seeds, unoiled (2 tablespoons = 1 serving)

Reduced-calorie margarine (2 tablespoons = 1 serving)

Reduced-fat salad dressing (2 tablespoons = 1 serving)

Salad dressing (1 tablespoon = 1 serving)

Trans-free margarine (1 tablespoon = 1 serving)

Optional Snacks

These snacks are all under 100 calories. Plus, they're filling and fun to eat.

Mini Babybel Light cheese—2 disks

Frozen fruit bar

Fudgesicle, 100 calorie bar

Granola bar, reduced sugar and fat

Microwave popcorn, light (4 cups)

Skinny Cow ice cream sandwich

Sugar-free pudding cup

String cheese—1 piece

Contour Foods on Cycle 3

In addition to all the Contour Foods you are now eating, on Cycle 3, you'll be eating even more, as I've listed here.

The Foods	How They Work
Additional whole grains and high-fiber breakfast cereals	These assist in burning fat around the abdominal area.
Soy milk	Soy contains natural substances that keep fat-storing hormones from depositing fat on thighs, hips, and stomach. (Soy can be highly allergenic to some people, however.)
Banana	Unless it is very ripe, a banana contains a type of starch that can help the body burn fat; it is called *resistant starch*, because it is a fiber that resists digestion.

Meal Planning Made Easy

Each day, for the next 17 days, you'll eat:

- Controlled portions of protein from an expanded list
- Liberal amounts of vegetables from an expanded list
- Two servings of natural starches from an expanded list
- Two servings of fruit from an expanded list
- One to two servings from probiotics, low-fat dairy, or dairy substitutes
- One serving of fat from an expanded list
- Optional snacks
- Optional daily serving of alcohol

Here is a typical day on the Achieve Cycle:

Breakfast

- ½ cup hot whole-grain cereal; or 2 eggs or 4 egg whites, prepared without oil; 1 *Dr. Mike's Power Cookie*; or 1 probiotic serving
- 1 fruit serving

Lunch

- Controlled portions of protein in the form of fish, shellfish, meat, or chicken or eggs; or vegetables plus 1 probiotic, dairy, or dairy substitute serving
- 1 serving natural starch
- Unlimited vegetables

Dinner

- Controlled portions of protein in the form of fish, shellfish, meat, or chicken or turkey
- Unlimited vegetables

Snacks

- 2nd fruit serving; or
- 2nd probiotic, dairy, or dairy substitute serving; or
- Food from optional snack list

Additional

- 1 serving (1 to 2 tablespoons of friendly fat to use on salads, vegetables, or for cooking)

SCIENCE SAYS: Liposuction Has Health Benefits

Thinking about getting liposuction? Talk to your doctor. Liposuction, like all procedures, has risks. But liposuction has been found to help reverse type 2 diabetes and reduce cholesterol.

As I have mentioned, obesity makes your body's cells resistant to insulin. Insulin is like an usher taking patrons to their seats in a theater, except that insulin takes glucose inside cells for energy. If cells are resistant to insulin, they don't open their doors to the hormone. The result is that sugar can't enter your cells, and your blood-sugar level rises. Liposuction seems to reverse that process. In a study at Brooklyn's SUNY Downstate Medical Center, a surgeon removed an average of 12 pounds of fat from 7 young women with type 2 diabetes. After the procedure, the women were no longer insulin resistant, and their blood-sugar levels dropped. The findings are intriguing. This was a small study, so it will be interesting to see if future studies into liposuction improve insulin resistance, too.

The other benefit of liposuction is this: Removing just 6 pounds of fat can lower your cholesterol level dramatically. That's what University of Salzburg researchers concluded. They think suctioning off just tiny amounts of fat changes a patient's metabolism for the better.

Although I prefer that you help your health the old-fashioned way—diet, exercise, determination, willpower, and dedication—these studies hold promise.

17 Sample Menus

Here are examples of how to build menus while on the Achieve Cycle. You can follow these exactly or create your own.

Wake-up Drink

Every morning, as soon as you rise, drink one 8-ounce cup of hot water. Squeeze a lemon into the cup; the lemon stimulates your digestive system. Drink at least six to seven more glasses of water by the end of the day, more if you can. The rate at which you burn calories drops if you're dehydrated. Also, if you're dehydrated, your body doesn't absorb nutrients properly.

Day 1

Breakfast

- 1 slice whole-wheat toast
- 1 poached, soft-boiled, or hard-boiled egg
- ½ grapefruit
- 1 cup green tea

Lunch

- Chicken Caesar salad: cut-up grilled chicken breast, 2 cups Romaine lettuce, other desired salad veggies, 2 tablespoons light Caesar dressing
- 1 slice whole-wheat toast
- 1 serving fresh fruit
- 1 cup green tea

Dinner

- Roasted pork tenderloin
- 1–2 cups baby spinach leaves with 2 tablespoons fat-free dressing
- 1 cup green tea

Snacks

- 1 probiotic, dairy, or dairy substitute serving
- 1 frozen fruit bar

Day 2

Breakfast

- 1 cup high-fiber cereal (i.e., Bran Buds or Fiber One)
- 1 cup skim, 1%, or soy milk or other dairy substitute
- 1 cup fresh berries
- 1 cup green tea

Lunch

- *Salad in a Sandwich*
- 10 baby carrots
- 1 cup green tea

Dinner

- *Oven Barbecued Chicken*
- Steamed vegetables such as asparagus, wax beans, broccoli, or cauliflower
- 1 cup green tea

Snacks

- 2nd fruit
- 1 Skinny Cow ice cream sandwich

Day 3

Breakfast

- 1 cup plain yogurt
- 1 sliced banana
- 1 slice cracked wheat toast
- Jam, 1 tablespoon (to mix with yogurt or on toast)
- 1 cup green tea

Lunch

- *Shrimp Cocktail with Avocado Dressing*
- *Pasta Caesar Salad*
- 1 cup green tea

Dinner

- *Salmon Lemonato*
- *Onion-Leek Soup*
- 1 cup green tea

Snacks

- *Mango Sorbet*
- 2nd probiotic, dairy, or dairy substitute serving

Day 4

Breakfast

- *Blueberry Griddle Cakes*
- 1 cup green tea

Lunch

- Broiled lean ground beef mixed with low-carb marinara sauce and served over ½ cup whole-wheat or gluten-free pasta
- 1–2 cups tossed mixed salad with 2 tablespoons reduced-fat dressing
- 1 cup green tea

Dinner

- 1 large bowl *Chicken Vegetable Soup*
- 1 cup green tea

Snacks

- 2nd fruit serving
- 2nd probiotic, dairy, or dairy substitute serving
- *Tropical Pistachio Pudding*

Day 5

Breakfast

- *South of the Border Scramble*
- 1 cup fresh berries
- 1 cup green tea

Lunch

- Tuna sandwich: tuna mixed with 1 tablespoon mayonnaise, chopped celery, and onion, served between two slices of whole-grain bread.
- 1 fresh pear
- 1 cup green tea

Dinner

- *Creamy Light Fettuccine Alfredo*
- Tossed side salad with fat-free dressing
- 1 cup green tea

Snacks

- Probiotic, dairy, or dairy substitute serving
- One 100-calorie Fudgesicle

Day 6

Breakfast

- 1 cup no-sugar-added fruit-flavored yogurt
- ½ cup *Lean Granola*
- 1 piece fresh fruit (i.e, 1 peach, ¼ cantaloupe, ½ grapefruit, or 1 orange)
- 1 cup green tea

Lunch

- *Avocado Stuffed with Scallops*
- Medium baked potato with 1 tablespoon fat-free sour cream, or ½ cup brown or Basmati rice
- 1 medium apple
- 1 cup green tea

Dinner

- *Spicy Beef Tips*
- Zucchini, sautéed with 1 tablespoon olive oil and Italian spices
- 1 cup green tea

Snack

- 2nd probiotic, dairy, or dairy substitute serving
- 1 frozen fruit bar

Day 7

Breakfast

- ½ cup low-fat or fat-free cottage cheese
- 1 cup pineapple chunks, fresh or canned, in their own juice
- 1 cup green tea

Lunch

- *Meat and Bean Burrito*
- *Tortilla Soup*, 1 bowl
- 1 cup green tea

Dinner

- *General Slim's Chicken*
- Steamed vegetables
- 1–2 cups tossed mixed salad with 2 tablespoons reduced-fat dressing
- 1 cup green tea

Day 8

Breakfast

- 1 *Dr. Mike's Power Cookie*
- 1 banana, sliced
- 1 cup nonfat or acidophilus milk
- 1 cup green tea

Lunch

- *Turkey Chili*
- 1 serving fresh fruit
- 1 cup green tea

Dinner

- Grilled salmon
- 1–2 cups tossed mixed salad with 2 tablespoons fat-free dressing
- 1 cup green tea

Snacks

- 1 probiotic, dairy, or dairy substitute serving
- 1 frozen fruit bar

Day 9

Breakfast

- *Breakfast Crisp*
- 6 ounces no-sugar-added fruit-flavored yogurt
- 1 cup fresh berries
- 1 cup green tea

Lunch

- *Super Salad*
- 1 medium baked potato, topped with 1 tablespoon fat-free sour cream, if desired
- 1 cup green tea

Dinner

- *Beef Fajita Salad*
- Steamed vegetable, such as asparagus, wax beans, broccoli, or cauliflower
- 1 cup green tea

Snacks

- 2nd fruit
- 1 Skinny Cow ice cream sandwich

Day 10

Breakfast

- ½ cup cooked oatmeal
- ½ grapefruit
- 1 cup green tea

Lunch

- *Salade Nicoise*
- 1 cup green tea

Dinner

- Baked turkey breast
- 1 medium baked sweet potato
- Green beans or other veggie, steamed
- 1 cup green tea

Snacks

- 2nd fruit serving
- 2nd probiotic, dairy, or dairy substitute serving

Day 11

Breakfast

- *Spanish Omelet*
- 1 medium apple or pear
- 1 cup green tea

Lunch

- Broiled lean ground beef mixed with low-carb marinara sauce and served over ½ cup whole-wheat or gluten-free pasta
- 1–2 cups tossed mixed salad with 2 tablespoons reduced-fat dressing
- 1 cup green tea

Dinner

- *Ceviche*
- Steamed green beans
- ½ cup acorn or butternut squash
- 1 cup green tea

Snacks

- 2nd fruit serving
- 2nd probiotic, dairy, or dairy substitute serving
- 1 Skinny Cow ice cream sandwich

Day 12

Breakfast

- 4 scrambled egg whites
- 1 slice Canadian bacon
- 1 cup melon balls
- 1 cup green tea

Lunch

- Chicken sandwich: grilled or baked chicken mixed with 1 tablespoon mayonnaise, chopped celery, and onion, served between two slices of whole-grain bread
- 1 fresh pear or other fruit in season
- 1 cup green tea

Dinner

- *Apricot-Glazed Lamb Chops*
- Steamed broccoli or cauliflower
- Cooked carrots
- 1 cup green tea

Snacks

- Probiotic, dairy, or dairy substitute serving
- One 100-calorie Fudgesicle

Day 13

Breakfast

- 1 cup no-sugar-added fruit-flavored yogurt
- 1 piece fresh fruit (i.e, 1 peach, ¼ cantaloupe, ½ grapefruit, or 1 orange)
- 1 cup green tea

Lunch

- Turkey sandwich: reduced-fat turkey, 1 slice reduced-fat Swiss cheese, mustard, lettuce, slice of tomato, between two slices of rye bread
- 1 medium apple
- 1 cup green tea

Dinner

- *Greek Chicken Stew*
- Zucchini, steamed
- 1 cup green tea

Snack

- 2nd probiotic, dairy, or dairy substitute serving
- 1 frozen fruit bar
- 1 cup green tea

Day 14

Breakfast

- 2 scrambled eggs
- 1 slice whole-grain toast
- 1 cup pineapple chunks, fresh or canned, in their own juice
- 1 cup green tea

Lunch

- *Lettuce Wraps*
- 1 cup green tea

Dinner

- *Bacon-Wrapped Scallops*
- *Light Fries*
- 1–2 cups tossed mixed salad with 2 tablespoons reduced-fat dressing
- 1 cup green tea

Day 15

Breakfast

- *Yogurt Smoothie*
- 1 slice whole-wheat toast
- 1 cup green tea

Lunch

- *Fried Fish*
- 1 serving fresh fruit
- 1 cup green tea

Dinner

- Roasted pork tenderloin
- *Brown Rice with Mushrooms*
- 1 cup green tea

Snacks

- 1 probiotic, dairy, or dairy substitute serving
- 1 frozen fruit bar

Day 16

Breakfast

- 1 cup high-fiber cereal (i.e., Bran Buds or Fiber One)
- 1 cup (8 oz.) skim, acidophilus, 1%, or soy milk or other dairy substitute
- 1 banana, sliced
- 1 cup green tea

Lunch

- *Salmon Burgers*
- Sliced tomato, drizzled with fat-free salad dressing
- 1 cup green tea

Dinner

- *Oven Barbecued Chicken*
- Steamed vegetables, such as asparagus, wax beans, broccoli, or cauliflower
- 1 cup green tea

Snacks

- 2nd fruit
- 1 Skinny Cow ice cream sandwich

Day 17

Breakfast

- 1 cup plain yogurt, mixed with 1 tablespoon sugar-free jam
- 1 cup fresh berries
- 1 cup green tea

Lunch

- *White Bean Hummus*, served on cucumber slices
- 1 cup green tea

Dinner

- Sirloin steak
- 1 medium baked potato with 1 tablespoon sour cream
- 1–2 cups tossed mixed salad with 1 tablespoon oil mixed with 2 tablespoons vinegar
- 1 cup green tea

Snacks

- *Banana Ice Cream*
- 2nd probiotic, dairy, or dairy substitute serving
- 1 fat-free pudding cup

Achieve Cycle Worksheet

It may help you to plan your meals using the following worksheet. Using the food lists, simply fill in what you will eat each day.

Breakfast

Protein or probiotic or low-fat dairy serving: _____

Starch serving: _____

Fruit serving: _____

Lunch

Protein: _____

Starch serving: _____

Vegetables: _____

Dinner

Protein serving: _____

Vegetables: _____

Snacks

2nd fruit serving: _____

2nd probiotic or low-fat dairy serving: _____

Optional snack: _____

Other

Friendly fat serving: _____

If You Have More Weight to Lose

At the end of Cycle 3, if you have additional weight to lose, you have several options:

- Return to Accelerate for 17 days, continue to Activate for 17 days, and follow with Achieve for 17 days; or
- Return to Activate for 17 days, and follow with Achieve for 17 days; or
- Continue with Achieve until you reach your goal weight.
- Use my Transitional Day Fast as a tool (see below).

Suggestion: If you are very close to your goal weight at the end of your first Achieve Cycle, it's best to return to the Accelerate Cycle for up to 17 days to reach your goal more quickly.

Your Optional Transitional Day Fast

Now that you've completed Cycle 3, you may want to opt for a Transitional Day Fast. Remember, it involves having three liquid meals on that day.

Breakfast

. . . .

Smoothie #1

1 cup unsweetened almond milk

½ cup plain low-fat yogurt

1 scoop vanilla whey powder

1 serving powdered fiber

½ cup crushed pineapple, canned in its own juice, drained

½ frozen banana

Place the ingredients in a blender, and blend until smooth. Tip: Blend the mixture for several minutes. This adds air to the smoothie, which will make you feel fuller. Makes 1 serving.

Lunch

If you're doing your Transitional Day Fast on a weekday, and you work, make your smoothie ahead of time and freeze it in a Ziploc bag. Take it to work and place it in a fridge. When lunch rolls around, it will be ready to drink.

. . . .

Smoothie #2

1 cup plain low-fat yogurt

⅓ cup unsweetened almond milk

1 cup frozen strawberries

1 serving vanilla whey protein powder

1 serving powdered fiber

Truvia, to taste

Place the ingredients in a blender, and blend until smooth. Freeze. Makes 1 serving.

Dinner

. . . .

Smoothie #3

1 cup unsweetened almond milk

½ cup frozen blueberries

Large handful fresh spinach

1 serving vanilla whey protein powder

1 teaspoon matcha

½ cup crushed ice

Truvia, to taste

Place the ingredients in a blender, and blend until smooth. Makes 1 serving.

Also, drink at least 8 cups of pure water, and enjoy 3 to 4 cups of green tea throughout the day.

• • • • • • • •

As we wrap up this cycle, think for a moment about how good it feels to slim down. Replacing those lost pounds should be newfound feelings of self-control, increased health and fitness, loose clothing, continual compliments, improved physical appearance, excitement, and an overall boost of pride. I know it hasn't been easy. But the accomplishment of losing weight will bring you true satisfaction—something a Happy Meal could never do.

SCIENCE SAYS: Snooze, You Lose (Weight)

Researchers are learning more about how critical sleep is to slimming down. Adequate sleep keeps important appetite and weight-loss hormones in balance so that you stay satisfied by what you eat. Lack of sleep throws off the levels of these hormones. Also, you are less likely to make healthy choices when you're tired.

Doctors have a long history of missing sleep, which may explain why many doctors are fat. Being sleep deprived goes back to our internship days when we sometimes had to stay up for 30 hours straight. Once I nodded off for a moment and almost strangled myself with my stethoscope.

If you don't have enough time to sleep at night, try to squeeze in a short nap during the day. Napping is good for losing weight, according to a study in the *American Journal of Physiology, Endocrinology, and Metabolism*. (That should be great news unless you have a newborn in the house, or you're apt to get fired for sleeping on the job.)

Anyway, the study measured hormone levels in 41 men and women who were part of a week-long sleep-deprivation experiment. Those participants who napped for two hours following a night without any sleep showed big drops in cortisol, a hormone activated by high levels of stress, and responsible for weight gain around the belly.

So, forget counting calories, start counting sheep.

MISTER M.D., CAN YOU PLEASE TELL ME

Why Can't I Drink Diet Soda on the 17 Day Diet?

Doesn't diet soda seem like a dieter's dream? You can swill down as much as you want, and none of it will glom onto your thighs, right? Wrong. These beverages are like spies, with a plot to make you put on pounds. Diet soda is flavored with noncaloric artificial sweeteners. Everyone knows this. But what everyone does not know is that the supersweet taste of artificial sweeteners triggers your cravings for real sugar and all the foods that contain it. The more diet soda you drink, the more you want real sugar. But, hey, I'm a fair guy. Have diet soft drinks in moderation, but concentrate more on drinking water, sparkling water, or seltzer, all of which keep cravings on an even keel without sparking a junk-food binge.

Review

- Cycle 3: Achieve is a more moderate, liberalized food plan that allows a wide range of healthy foods, eaten in proper portions for continued weight loss.

- Weight loss may slow down during Cycle 3, but you can speed it up by: increasing your aerobic exercise; not eating carbohydrates of any type past 2 p.m., including more Contour Foods; using my Transitional Day Fast, and avoiding optional alcohol.

- The purpose of Cycle 3 is to help you achieve good eating habits.

8

Cycle 4: Arrive

You made it! Applause, everyone!

You started the 17 Day Diet, and you decided you'd do it for just 17 days. That worked wonders, so then you committed to another 17 days, and another. You felt so good about yourself, and proud of your achievement, that you decided to go right to your goal. By stringing those 17 day cycles together, you reached that goal.

You have overcome your weight problem! Now it's time to keep the pounds off, but how? With what I call the Arrive Cycle, because you've *arrived* at your goal weight. This is a huge, important accomplishment, something many people fail to do. Now, the important thing is that you stay at this weight.

At this point in the book, I have to be really, really honest, and talk about a big, unmentionable thing, something no one wants to admit.

You will always be on some kind of diet.

You will not be able to return to your former eating and nonexercising habits and keep the weight off, because those very habits—like eating your way into a gallon of Rocky Road ice cream and being inactive—created the weight in the first place. So, you've always got to diet, if you want to maintain this weight loss. Maintenance plans, in the dieting vernacular, really mean nothing more than following another diet.

Whaddaya mean, I've got to diet forever?

Yes, it's true, you've always got to watch your weight. Sorry. Keeping weight off is a bear, a big, hungry, growling one. Once a dieter, always a dieter.

Got that? Okay, so at least let's have some fun doing it.

What I propose as a keep-it-off strategy is weekends off.

Let's face it: Weekends have never been good for diets. You earn a promotion on Friday, so you eat to celebrate. Or you go to the movies on Friday or Saturday, and you eat a jumbo carton of popcorn. Or you go to a party, and eat your way through the snack table. The whole weekend is a problem and your behavior changes, and not always for the better. Would thick layers of duct tape around your mouth help?

Taking weekends off allows you to splurge a bit, making it easier to get back on track on Monday. Most people can be pretty disciplined Monday through Thursday, choosing meals carefully, getting in some exercise, and seeing decent results on the scale. The Arrive Cycle capitalizes on these normal rhythms of life and builds a *livable* maintenance plan around them.

In a nutshell, here's how you keep weight off: Stay strict during the week, then enjoy yourself more over the weekend. Most people do this to lose weight. I advise that you do it to keep weight off.

I'm giving you the best diet present you can have. You still eat a calorie-controlled diet during the week then, on weekends, have what you like. You take off plenty of pounds, and you'll keep that weight off. Plus, you'll never get discouraged using my weekend principle.

The Arrive Cycle is metabolically strategic, too. You can control your weight efficiently because you're shocking your metabolism back into action. Why? Because you're following five days of controlled eating, followed by two days of increased calories. By adding calories to your meals—with hamburgers, bread, ice cream, wine, cheesecake, you name it—you're speeding up your metabolism. Then, when your metabolism is roaring like a furnace, you get back to your diet on Monday, burning calories faster than ever. Basically, the Arrive Cycle keeps your metabolism guessing, so it never has a chance to go into hibernation. Since your metabolism is now well trained, due to better eating habits and digestive health, a few cheat treats on the weekend will not have an adverse effect.

The Arrive Cycle is not a free-for-all. You're allowed some of your favorite foods in moderation. For example, Friday night: A restaurant meal with a cocktail or two. Saturday: A slice or two of pizza for lunch or dinner, plus one dessert. Sunday: Pancakes with maple syrup.

A good rule of thumb to follow while stabilizing your weight is to enjoy no more than three favorite meals each weekend.

I call this *strategic cheating*.

I must add a warning: If the only time you aren't putting things in your mouth is when you're asleep, you may have an eating disorder, or a history of one. If so, this way of eating is not for you. However, 99 percent of dieters who follow the 17 Day Diet are ready and motivated to live the Arrive Cycle. I'll give you some supereasy strategies to make sure that strategic cheating on weekends doesn't turn into pigging out during the week.

Breathe a sigh of relief. Life is about to get normal, with you locked in at a normal, healthy, beautiful weight.

I Did It the 17 Day Way! Marjorie

It has been a year since I purchased Dr. Mike Moreno's book, and it has changed my life. I am a 45-year-old mother of three. With each pregnancy, I gained weight and kept on an extra 10 pounds afterward. After my third child was a toddler, I joined a local gym and started exercising a few times a week, thinking it would help me lose weight. It didn't. One night, I was browsing the Kindle store, and I happened upon *The 17 Day Diet*. I was intrigued and thought "I can do anything for 17 days!"

Dr. Mike's formula for weight loss became my new way of life. I won't lie: The first 17 days were tough! But, I stuck with it and lost weight steadily, exercising almost every day. Running became my new passion and, since May 2013, I have run in three different 10K races: I have never been more fit.

My total weight loss was 43 pounds, and I am happy to report that I am keeping it off. I can never go back to the way I used to eat, but I don't want to! This new me is much healthier and happier and also many sizes smaller! Thank-you, Dr. Mike, for a simple and effective diet that works. I recommend your diet to everyone!

Start the Arrive Cycle

The Arrive Cycle is unique in that it helps you keep your weight off, while letting you enjoy yourself and eat freely from your favorite foods on weekends.

Basically, the Arrive Cycle works like this:

- Monday breakfast through Friday lunch: Enjoy meal plans from one of your favorite Cycles: Accelerate, Activate, or Achieve.

- Friday dinner through Sunday dinner: Enjoy your favorite foods and meals in moderation over the weekend.

- Enjoy no more than one to three favorite meals over the weekend. Do not binge. Eat slowly and enjoy your food.

- If desired, enjoy alcoholic drinks in moderation over the weekend (1 to 2 daily): 1½ oz. hard liquor, 5 oz. wine, or 12 oz. beer.

- You may include soups in your daily menus, as long as they are broth-based. Avoid soups made with milk or cream. Having soup prior to a meal will help curb your appetite and help you feel full.

- As one of your fruit servings, you may substitute fruit juice (unsweetened), but no more than ¾ cup per serving.

- Feel free to enjoy 1 cup of vegetable juice as a snack.

- Continue to use condiments in moderation. Choose nonfat, low-calorie seasonings, such as reduced-fat dressings, spices, herbs, lemon or lime juice, vinegar, and hot sauce.

- Exercise on weekends, as well as weekdays.

- Each Monday, I'd like you to renew your commitment to yourself and to your new incredible body. Do this, and you'll control your eating week by week, with a strategy that'll guarantee success.

The Arrive Cycle Lifestyle

Let me give you an example of how this cycle works in real life. Mary lost 30 pounds on the 17 Day Diet. To keep those pounds off, she follows the Accelerate Cycle Monday through Friday. For the weekends, she plans meals at which she will enjoy her favorite foods. Whatever she wants the most, she lets herself have on those designated weekend days. Planning is key; it is far better than spontaneous splurges.

"It was important for me to know that I had these little treats coming," Mary says, "but it was even more important to know that I would get right back on the diet on Monday, and I always did."

Here's a look at Mary's typical week.

Monday

Breakfast

- 6 ounces plain low-fat yogurt, mixed with 1 cup berries, or other fruit (chopped)
- 1 cup green tea

Lunch

- A large salad with lots of cleansing vegetables and some flaxseed dressing
- 1 medium apple
- 1 cup green tea

Dinner

- Plenty of grilled or baked salmon
- Liberal amounts of cleansing vegetables, steamed or raw
- 1 cup green tea

Snacks

- 6 ounces no-sugar-added fruit-flavored yogurt or 1 cup plain low-fat yogurt
- Baby carrots

Tuesday

Breakfast

- 2 scrambled eggs
- 1 medium pear or other fruit in season
- 1 cup green tea

Lunch

- Broiled hamburger
- Sliced or stewed tomatoes
- 1 cup green tea

Dinner

- A stir-fry of vegetables (broccoli, onions, julienne carrots, red pepper, etc.), and chicken strips with 1 tablespoon of olive oil
- 1 cup green tea

Snacks

- 1 cup fresh berries with 6 ounces of yogurt
- 1 bowl of low-fat, low-sodium chicken broth with miso (low-sodium)

Wednesday

Breakfast

- ½ cup Breakstone LiveActive cottage cheese
- 1 medium orange
- 1 cup green tea

Lunch

- Tuna on a generous bed of salad greens with fat-free salad dressing
- 1 medium apple
- 1 cup green tea

Dinner

- Grilled chicken breast
- Steamed asparagus
- Side salad drizzled with 1 tablespoon olive or flaxseed oil, mixed with 2 tablespoons balsamic vinegar and seasonings
- 1 cup green tea

Snacks

- 6 ounces plain low-fat yogurt
- Raw, cut-up veggies

Thursday

Breakfast

- 2 hard-boiled or poached eggs
- ½ grapefruit or other fresh fruit in season
- 1 cup green tea

Lunch

- Baked turkey breast
- Tomatoes, sliced or stewed, drizzled with 1 tablespoon flaxseed oil
- 6 ounces yogurt
- 1 cup green tea

Dinner

- Grilled salmon
- Steamed green beans
- 1 cup green tea

Snacks

- 1 medium orange
- 1 cup acidophilus milk or 6 ounces yogurt

Friday

Breakfast

- *Kefir Smoothie*
- 1 cup green tea

Lunch

- Grilled chicken tossed with reduced-fat salad dressing, served over a generous bed of lettuce
- 1 cup green tea

Dinner out with Friends

- Vegetable lasagna
- Tossed salad with blue cheese dressing
- Two 5-ounce glasses of wine
- Tiramisu, 1 serving

Snacks

- 1 medium apple
- 6 ounces plain low-fat yogurt

Saturday

Breakfast

- 2 scrambled eggs
- ½ grapefruit
- 1 cup green tea

Lunch

- Grilled salmon on a generous bed of lettuce with reduced-fat salad dressing
- 1 cup green tea

Dinner at a Steakhouse

- Grilled rib eye steak
- Caesar side salad with dressing
- 1 medium baked sweet potato
- Two 5 ounce glasses of wine

Snacks

- 1 cup fresh berries
- 1 cup acidophilus milk or 6 ounces plain low-fat yogurt

Sunday

Brunch

- Blueberry waffles with 2 tbsp. syrup
- Turkey sausage, 2 patties
- 1 cup orange juice

Dinner

- Grilled chicken breast
- Steamed broccoli
- *Mom's Apple Pie*
- 1 cup green tea

Snacks

- 6 ounces no-sugar-added fruit-flavored yogurt or 1 cup plain low-fat yogurt
- Baby carrots, raw

Analyze Mary's week. Note that it exemplifies a reasonable, moderate way of eating. She sticks to her diet during the week, but gives herself a little splurge room on the weekends. "I love Italian food and good wine, and I get to enjoy it on the weekends. Come Monday, I just go right back to the 17 Day Diet principles," she says.

Mary planned her three favorite meals for the weekend. The rest of the time, she ate prudently, following the Accelerate Cycle. Mary walks briskly most days of the week and always on the weekends. There's no way she's going to regain any weight. Sometimes, she even loses weight.

The Arrive Cycle is about being healthier and smarter about your selections and not pigging out. If you want to have some fried chicken on the weekends, you can do it. You're compensating by having healthier foods through the week. All is not lost. You don't really have to eliminate those foods. It's more about moderation and how to incorporate those foods in your diet.

As Mary did, all you have to do is follow your favorite cycle, essentially five days a week, then take weekends off. And make sure you exercise.

Arrive Cycle Strategies

I want to give you a bagful of Arrive Cycle tricks to keep you going. In my experience with patients, here's what works for lasting weight control.

Observe the 5-Pound Stop Signal

On the Arrive Cycle, weigh yourself on the weekends. Anytime you see the scale register three to five pounds over your weight goal, go right back on your favorite Cycle, Accelerate, Activate, or Achieve, on Monday. Note: You'll always get back to your normal weight faster by resuming the Accelerate Cycle. If, for some reason, you've gained a great deal of weight (perhaps by being on vacation), your solution is to start the 17 Day Diet from the beginning and progress through all Cycles. And definitely use my Transitional Day Fast between Cycles to help.

Oftentimes, busy lives take over after the diet, and people do not notice even large gains in weight. It's much easier to lose three pounds than 20. Plus, studies show that people who stop weighing themselves regain weight. Don't let that happen to you!

Be a Breakfast Lover

On most diets, people starve themselves in the morning, so that they can eat more for lunch and dinner. This doesn't work. Eat breakfast. Heck, any time someone tells you to eat, you really should listen!

You must eat breakfast. You say you don't feel that hungry in the morning? Okay, but eat anyway, because research shows that eating first thing will make you feel more satisfied throughout the entire day, and you'll consume fewer calories, all told. Even on weekends. What's more, I've personally found that most people who skip breakfast become ravenous by 10:30 in the morning and often find themselves eating whatever is on hand, even if it's really fattening junk food.

Get on Good Terms with Salad

Have a salad when you dine out or eat at home. According to a study at Penn State University, starting dinner with a large salad may help lower the number of calories you'll consume at that meal. What's the best salad to have? That's a no-brainer: a salad of mostly greens and veggies, topped with one tablespoon of light dressing.

Make Healthier Substitutes

Try to eat reduced-fat, reduced-sugar foods. These include:

- Mustard instead of mayo on sandwiches
- Skim milk instead of the whole stuff
- Butter-flavored cooking spray (to spritz on a baked potato, for example, or for sautéing)
- Salsa for dipping
- Reduced-sugar ketchup or steak sauce
- Fat-free, sugar-free ice cream and frozen treats
- Fat-free sour cream on baked potatoes instead of butter and sour cream
- Fat-free or reduced-calorie salad dressings
- Grilled chicken or turkey sandwiches instead of burgers at fast-food joints

    Every little bit helps.

Exercise Portion Control

What's the major dietary blunder of the last 10 years? Ginormous portions of rice and pasta and boulder-sized potatoes and yams. Large portions and rich food in restaurants are a major source of extra calories for Americans, a fact not likely to change soon. (More on this in chapter 8.) It's important to recognize this and to continue to choose well when dining out, and control portion sizes. Pay attention to portion sizes, and don't reach for seconds.

LEAN 17: 17 Foods that Increase Fullness and Tame Hunger

You don't need appetite suppressants, other than the following appetite-suppressing foods. Plan your menus to incorporate these foods, and you'll control your weight naturally:

1. Almonds
2. Apples
3. Beef, lean
4. Carrots
5. Whole-grain cereals
6. Chicken
7. Chickpeas
8. Eggs
9. Fish
10. Lentils
11. Prunes
12. Red hot peppers
13. Rye bread
14. Spinach
15. Walnuts
16. Whey protein smoothies
17. Yogurt

Source: Rebello, C. J., et al. 2013. Dietary strategies to increase satiety. *Advances in Food and Nutrition Research* 69:105–182.

Move It, Keep It Off

I said you could eat more food on the weekend, but I'm also saying you should burn off more of that food. Think about it: The weekend is when you have more time, usually, to exercise, so take advantage of your free time. Get in at least an hour of intense, heart-pumping exercise on both Saturday and Sunday. If you do this, it will be a cinch to keep your weight off. Exercise is one thing that really keeps you thin and fit.

Find ways to sneak in lifestyle activity, too, especially on weekends. Yard work is a great example. I cringe when I see people on riding mowers, the kind used by farmers to clear large tracts of land. Now people are using it to mow a patch of grass the size of a bath mat. Lawn mowing is great exercise, but only if you push the mower. It burns 387 calories an hour!

Here's what other weekend chores burn per hour:

LEAN 17: 17 Weekend Chores That Incinerate Calories (per hour)

1.	Watering lawn and garden by hand	102
2.	Cleaning, dusting	176
3.	Moderate housework	246
4.	Carpentry, general	246
5.	Plumbing	246
6.	Gardening	281
7.	Bagging grass	281
8.	Raking lawn	303
9.	Weeding or planting a garden	317
10.	Painting	317
11.	Cleaning gutters	352
12.	Chopping wood, slowly	362
13.	Remodeling	387
14.	Shoveling snow	422
15.	Moving heavy objects	528
16.	Farming, baling hay, cleaning barn	563
17.	Trimming trees	633

Avoid Overboard Syndrome

Never binge. Translated: No pig-outs. No stuffing your face until it grows to the size of a basketball. Get your eating under control. Decide that this way of eating is going to change.

Make lists of trouble foods that might make you binge. Deep down, you know what these foods are, so it's best to not include them in your weekend treat meals.

Plan your week's meals in advance, so that you're programming your brain and stomach to expect food. It will help you stop eating out of habit.

Stick to one of the cycles during the week; enjoy your favorite foods on the weekends. But use your head. Go ahead and include pizza in your nutrition plan—just choose a single slice, not the whole pie! Maintain that consistency, and you'll be thin for life.

No More Guilt Trips

On the Arrive Cycle, there's no need to struggle with the dieter's mentality that one bad or good deed will either break or make your weight loss efforts. You have permission to indulge, as long as it's planned and doesn't spin out of control into weekdays. You're in control; food is not in control of you. Remembering this will help you bounce back into wise eating on Monday.

And if you ever fall off the diet horse? Pick yourself up and get back in the saddle. Don't whip yourself with guilt. I don't expect perfection, but I expect progress. Simply return to the program at the very next meal. You'll feel better about yourself. And congratulate yourself for the strength of spirit it takes to get going again.

Stay Focused

I often repeat the phrase, "If you always do what you always did, you'll always get what you always got." This mantra will help you remember that if you revert to old habits, then say *hello* to the return of pounds. Remind yourself of how great you look. Keep pictures of your new body around where you can see them: on your fridge, on your bathroom mirror, at your desk, on your dashboard, among other places. Look at them when you want to eat something fattening, skip your workout, or zip through a drive-through. Also, list reasons that you want never to get fat again and put them next to your slim pictures. Also, wear tight clothing (it should fit well now), so that you stop eating when you feel fat. That's a little trick one of my patients taught me.

The truth about the Arrive Cycle is that it involves more than following a diet. It's about making a permanent change in behavior. This is a lifestyle change, a new way of living. You can now manage a lifetime of good nutrition, enjoy food, and keep fat from creeping back on.

Review

- The Arrive Cycle is the weight-stabilization part of the 17 Day Diet.
- It provides a realistic way for you to manage your food and lifestyle.
- The foundational principle underlying the Arrive Cycle is to enjoy meal plans from one of your favorite cycles—Accelerate, Activate, or Achieve—from Monday through Friday lunch. Then Friday dinner through Sunday dinner enjoy your favorite foods and meals in moderation.
- Enjoy no more than one to three favorite meals over the weekend. Do not binge. Eat slowly and enjoy your food.

LEAN 17: So-Called Healthy Foods That Will Make You Fat

Some foods with healthy reputations are actually worse for your weight than you might think. Take a look.

Food Fattening Factor

1. **Dried Fruit.** Cup for cup, dried fruit has tons more calories than the fresh kind, because it has been dehydrated and is much denser. Fresh grapes, for example, have 60 calories per cup, while raisins have 460.

2. **Granola.** It's loaded with good-for-you nuts and oats, but is also loaded with oil and sugar for more flavor. One bowl racks up around 500 calories. Try low-fat granola instead.

3. **Bran Muffin.** Most bran muffins are basically just a round piece of cake. One muffin can weigh in at about 20 grams of fat, 420 calories, and 34 grams of sugar.

4. **Bagel.** Many bagels weigh four to five ounces. At 80 calories per ounce, that's a 320- to 400-calorie hunk of bread. Stick to small whole-wheat bagels.

5. **Half-and-Half.** It seems harmless; after all, you put so little in your coffee or tea. But a few spoonfuls per cup of joe two or three times per day quickly turn into 200 or more calories, plus the same amount of fat as a big pat of butter.

6. **Flavored Coffee.** Drinks at coffeehouses will sabotage your diet faster than you can say Frappuccino. Some of these items top out at 700 calories per serving.

7. **Bottled Tea.** Most store-bought brands are souped up with sugar or honey. Oh, and one bottle can contain two or more servings, bringing the calorie count to almost 200, similar to a can of soda.

8. **Rice Cakes.** These light snacks are fat-free and low in calories, but they're also completely lacking in fiber or protein—ingredients that can tame your hunger. That means downing two or three won't do anything but add more calories to your daily total and leave you craving something with substance.

9. **Juice.** This is basically sugar and calories. A 16-ounce bottle of orange juice or apple juice has 55 grams of carbohydrate, the equivalent of five slices of bread. And most of that is sugar: a whopping 12 spoonfuls of it.

10. **Fat-Free Frozen Dessert.** The label might say it's as little as 60 calories for a small cup, but lab tests on these frozen delights say otherwise: around 270 calories is more like it.

11. **Reduced-Fat Cookies.** Three of these will give you 150 calories. But get this: Three regular chocolate-chip cookies are 160, just 10 measly calories more.

12. **Energy Bars.** The average candy bar has 250 calories; so does the average energy bar. Energy bars are candy bars incognito, disguised by a few added vitamins (which you're better off getting from fruit). Personally, I'd rather have a Snickers.

13. **Energy Drinks.** The labels say they contain various herbs, minerals, and the amino acid taurine, specially designed to boost your energy. However, if you look at the ingredients, they're mostly caffeine and sugar, making them hardly more than high-priced soft drinks.

14. **Diet Drinks.** The artificial sweeteners they contain make it harder for people to regulate their calorie intake. Sweet tastes tell the brain a lot of calories are about to be consumed. When that doesn't happen, you may eat more to compensate.

15. **Taco Salad.** One of these can weigh in at more than 900 calories (that's if you eat the hard-to-resist shell). Try my recipe for taco salad instead.

16. **Trail Mix.** Just three little tablespoons of this snack packs around 140 calories. Most people gobble down much more than that, making this a very high-calorie snack.

PART THREE

· ·

Special Considerations

9

The 17 Day Cultural Diet

I look Italian. Most people think I am Italian, except of course for Italians who think I'm from South America. My ancestry is Mexican; I was born and raised in the United States. Because of my origins, I'm able to relate to patients from many different cultures and, of course, because I speak Spanish, I can communicate with my Hispanic patients without an interpreter.

Language issues are important in medicine. A lot of people who seek medical help can't speak English, and sometimes find themselves getting the wrong treatment, which can turn out to be both costly and embarrassing. We had a man once who was about to be treated for back problems. However, he didn't have back problems, he had constipation. He was trying to refer to his "backside," but the nurse thought he meant "back." Or maybe he was too embarrassed to point to that part of his body.

In the nutrition area, I feel strongly that many people, due to their heritage, are not getting adequate nutritional counseling to lose weight. This is a big problem. When people come to the United States from other countries, they leave their traditional foods behind and adopt the Americanized diet that is loaded with refined carbohydrates, sugar, and bad fats—often with life-threatening consequences. Hispanics, for example, tend to develop type 2 diabetes as early as their thirties and forties. That's about 10 years earlier than most of the population. This tendency is set off by weight gain, a sedentary lifestyle, and smoking. Heart disease is another risk. Unfortunately, much of the diet advice that Hispanics get in the United States doesn't square with their beliefs about food or their cultural practices. The same is true for many other cultures.

I can't solve that problem in one chapter, but I'm going to give you a list of foods from your culture that you can eat on all four Cycles of the 17 Day Diet, if your heritage is Hispanic, Asian, Mediterranean, Indian, or Middle Eastern.

Hispanic Cuisine

As I know, fried food, grease, and salt are three of the basic food groups in the typical Hispanic diet—and what triggers so many life-threatening diseases in Hispanic men, women, and children.

The good news is that, if you are Hispanic, you don't have to kick your ethnic favorites out of your diet. You just need to tweak the ingredients and the prep. Let's look at the food lists.

Cycle 1: Accelerate

Stick to the lists of approved foods, but add these cultural selections.

Lean Proteins

Ceviche (white fish marinated in lemon juice with diced tomatoes, onions, chili peppers, and cilantro)

Red snapper (*huachinango*)

Cleansing Vegetables

Concentrate on traditional favorites such as tomatoes, onion, summer squash, cauliflower, garlic, green beans, and chilies (literally hundreds of varieties); tomatillos; and cilantro

Cycle 2: Activate

Stick to the list of approved foods, but add these cultural selections:

Lean Proteins

Reduced-fat chorizo

Goat meat

Natural Starches

Focus on all varieties of beans and legumes

Use brown rice instead of white

Calabaza

Yucca (cassava root or manioc)

Arracacha

Yautia

Plantains

Cycle 3: Achieve

Stick to the list of approved foods, but add in these cultural selections:

Lean Protein

Introduce the Hispanic-style cheese, *queso fresco*, or "fresh cheese" as a protein. It contains fewer calories, and less fat and cholesterol than other popular cheeses such as cheddar or processed cheese products. It's not fake cheese either, thank goodness. My idea of hell is a place where Mexican food is made with artificial cheese.

Natural Starches

Low-carb tortillas

Corn (maize) tortillas

Bolillos (sourdough bread)

Cleansing Vegetables

Chayote

Jicama

Nopales

General Tips

- Many Mexican dishes such as beans, tortillas, and Spanish rice are healthy sources of carbohydrates. Beans are loaded with fat-fighting, digestion-friendly fiber. However, it is necessary to depart from tradition when it comes to frying or refrying. No more frying foods in lard and other fat. Try boiling or sautéing with vegetable cooking spray instead.

- Try preparing refried beans with less oil (use olive oil, not lard), or put them through a food processor and sauté them in a pan that has been coated with vegetable cooking spray.

- Scale back your intake of sour cream (try Greek yogurt instead). Or use salsa or pico de gallo to top your entrees.

- Reduce fat by using a variety of cooking sprays—and for much more than just sautéing. Try butter-flavored sprays for softening or baking tortillas, or olive oil sprays on grilled vegetables, fish, or poultry.

- Use herbs and chilies in place of fats and oils.

- Use low-fat or fat-free cream cheeses. Fat-free cream cheese or low-fat ricotta lends a creamy texture to beans and sauces. Combine fat-free cream cheese and low-fat buttermilk to make a sour cream sauce. Avoid nonfat sour cream, which tends to have an offensive taste.

- Use low-fat cheeses in small amounts. They are tastier when mixed with highly flavored ingredients like chilies, spices, and salsas.

- Instead of cooking tortillas in oil or other fat, brown them on the griddle, then oven bake them a few minutes to heat through.

- Focus on eating simply prepared dishes flavored with traditional seasonings minus high-carb, high-fat sauces. Salsa is another favorite made from finely diced tomatoes, onions, and chili peppers. This green or red chili sauce adds spice to a meal but not many calories. Many Hispanics are not used to eating foods without grease or salt. But, with the right spices, the tastes can almost be duplicated.

Mediterranean Cuisine

There's actually no one Mediterranean diet, when you consider that at least 16 countries border the Mediterranean Sea. The region's cuisines include

Italian, Greek, and Spanish. Diets vary among all these countries and also among regions within a country (such as northern Italian food with its white sauces and southern Italian food with its red sauces). However, the cuisines of Mediterranean countries have several things in common:

- Lots of fruits and vegetables
- Inclusion of bread and other cereals, potatoes, beans, nuts, and seeds
- Emphasis on olive oil as an important monounsaturated fat source (Monounsaturated fat doesn't raise blood-cholesterol levels the way saturated fat does.)
- Low-to-moderate consumption of red meat, fish. and poultry
- Low-to-moderate consumption of cheese and yogurt
- Moderate consumption of red wine

Sounds healthy. Does a Mediterranean-style diet follow the 17 Day Diet recommendations?

Close, but not exactly. In general, the diets of Mediterranean peoples are higher in calories from fat. This is thought to contribute to the increasing obesity in these countries, which is becoming a concern.

For the most part, the Mediterranean diet is fresh and flavored with garlic, onions, fresh herbs, tomatoes, and other vegetables. It is, therefore, enormously rich in antioxidants.

Most of the foods on the 17 Day Diet are found in Mediterranean cuisine. Here are a few to add.

Cycle 1: Accelerate

Stick to the lists of approved foods, but add these cultural selections:

Cleansing Vegetables

Broccoli rabe

Fennel

Italian flat-leaf parsley

Sugar-free marinara sauce (½ cup = 1 serving)

Cycle 2: Activate

Adhere to the list of acceptable foods, but add these cultural selections:

Natural Starches

Orzo

Polenta

Tabouli (Crushed wheat kernels that have been boiled and mixed
with ingredients such as veggies, parsley, and mint, and dressed
with olive oil and lemon juice)

Cycle 3: Achieve

Stick to the list of acceptable foods, but add these cultural selections:

Natural Starches

White whole-grain, whole-wheat, and multigrain flatbreads

Whole-grain Italian bread

General Tips

- Serve hot grilled chicken on a bed of steamed broccoli rabe sprinkled
  with lemon juice and pepper.
- Cook liberally with canned tomatoes. Cooked tomatoes are higher in
  beneficial antioxidants, such as cancer-fighting lycopene, than raw
  tomatoes.
- Avoid fattening butter sauces, and stick with tomato-based sauces,
  such as marinara. The calorie count will be lower.
- Try sliced fennel sautéed over a little olive oil until translucent. Add
  cannellini beans, and top with a piece of salmon. Sprinkle with
  chopped Italian flat-leaf parsley for a great Activate Cycle meal.
- Use whole-grain pastas, spaghetti squash, or shirataki noodles (low-
  carb pasta) in place of regular pasta.

- Reduce the oil when making hummus and baba ghannoush, or skip it altogether.
- Dip sliced cucumbers, rather than bread, in hummus.
- Use whole-grain pita bread over white bread.
- For a nutritious, high-fiber, low-fat lunch, try whole-wheat pita bread stuffed with Greek salad.
- Heart-healthy main dishes include shish kebabs, souvlaki, or plaki (fish baked or broiled with garlic and tomato sauce). Dolmas (stuffed vegetables or grape leaves) make an excellent choice because they are usually steamed or baked.
- For condiments: Use certain spices that are popular in the Mediterranean diet, such as oregano, parsley, and basil, as well as healthy veggies like onions and garlic.

Asian Cuisine

Asian diets are associated with the best life expectancy in the world. The longevity can be chalked up to a healthy, low-fat diet. This dietary regimen is linked to a lower frequency of heart attacks and strokes than we see in other countries. Asians also eat their meals at regular times, chew their food well, take in lots of fiber through vegetables and fruits, and drink green tea frequently. Here's how to adapt the 17 Day Diet to Asian dietary standards.

Cycle 1: Accelerate

Stick to the lists of approved foods, but add these cultural selections:

Cleansing Vegetables

Arame, a form of kelp, best known in Japanese cuisine

Bamboo shoots

Bean sprouts

Bok choy

Chinese broccoli

Dulce, sea lettuce (used in many international cuisines)

Lily pods

Long beans (an Asian vegetable similar to green beans)

Nori, an edible seaweed commonly used as a wrap for sushi

Pea pods

Snow peas

Cycle 2: Activate

Stick to the list of approved foods, but add these cultural selections:

Lean Protein

Tofu, all varieties

Organic bison meat

Natural Starches

Edamame

Substitute brown rice for white rice

Cycle 3: Achieve

Natural Starches

Add the following starches (1 serving = ½ cup):

- Soba noodles: Japanese noodles made from buckwheat flour.
- Ramen noodles: Thin noodles very popular in Asian cuisine.
- Rice noodles: As the name suggests, these noodles, which are used throughout Southeast Asia, are made with rice flour.
- Chinese wheat noodles: A variety of noodles made from wheat and sometimes eggs.
- Udon noodles: A type of wheat-flour noodle popular in Japanese cuisine.

- Miracle noodles: Here is a way to have your noodles and eat them too. Made with a special type of fiber called *glucomannan*, these noodles have no carbs, no gluten, and no calories. They're delicious too and help keep blood sugar stable. You can enjoy them in any dish that uses Asian-type noodles, and even in chicken-noodle soup. Miracle noodles come in a variety of styles, including angel hair and ziti. There is a rice version too. Check this product out at www.miraclenoodle.com.

General Tips

- Boil, grill, steam, or lightly stir-fry seafood, chicken, vegetable, and tofu dishes—healthy techniques that require minimal fat.
- Steam foods such as fish or veggies in a multilayered bamboo basket. You can prepare several different dishes in one pot in about 10 to 15 minutes. As a bonus, veggies, fish, and other foods stay flavorful and nutritious when steamed.
- Don't deep fry. Use a skillet and spray it with vegetable cooking spray as needed. You'll end up getting the same effect without all the fattening oil.
- Avoid making thick sauces laced with fat and sodium.
- Substitute tofu in recipes that call for eggs.
- Substitute turkey for beef whenever possible. Turkey has a lot less saturated fat than red meat. Eat more fish than meat.
- Enjoy green tea, recommended on the 17 Day Diet. It contains powerful antioxidants that do more for your health than you can imagine: It normalizes cholesterol levels, protects your heart, boosts your immunity, perhaps even annihilates cancer and fat cells.
- For condiments, experiment with exotic fat-free flavors: light soy sauce, fish sauce, oyster sauce, black bean sauce, miso (fermented Japanese bean paste that is a probiotic), seaweed, chilies, wasabi (Japanese horseradish paste), kimchi (a Korean condiment made from pickled cabbage that is a probiotic), curries (favored in Thailand), garlic, scallions, ginger, lemon grass, basil, and cilantro.
- What about fortune cookies? Strictly an American invention.

Indian Cuisine

Generally, Indian meals are healthy and well balanced. They're full of antioxidant-rich vegetables; meat, fish, and chicken. Vegetarian dishes are often the centerpiece of meals, too. Generally, the unique spices used in Indian dishes add flavor without fat. Here's how to adapt the 17 Day Diet to Indian dietary standards.

Cycle 1: Accelerate

Cleansing Vegetables

Vegetables such as curry, coriander, or mint leaves

Cycle 2: Activate

Natural Starches

Basmati rice
Red lentils

Cycle 3: Achieve

Natural Starches

Chapatis (unleavened flatbread made from whole-wheat flour)
Any type of flatbread made from white whole-grain, whole-wheat, and multigrain flour

General Tips

- Vegetable curries, salads, shredded vegetables, and lentils make great high-fiber side dishes.
- Try tandoori chicken or fish for a low-fat meal; both are yummy.
- Use yogurt, too, as a low-fat substitute for cream and a thickener for curries.

- Replace ghee, a clarified butter, with olive oil or flaxseed oil. There is also a cholesterol-free ghee.

- Spices are an integral part of Indian cooking and alleviate the need to cook with a lot of fat. Some of the best spices for digestion include ginger, cumin, coriander, fennel, and cinnamon. Turmeric is pervasive in Indian cooking and is prized as a superspice because it stimulates digestion, improves liver function, and strengthens immunity.

Middle Eastern Cuisine

Although Middle Eastern cooking may seem exotic to Westerners, its presence is felt today in our own kitchens. When we cook with oranges, pistachios, spinach, or saffron, for example, we use foods that originated in the region around Persia, now called Iran. When we use basil, cilantro, cumin, and caraway, we are drawing on an age-old tradition of meatless cooking adopted by the Middle East from the empires of Sumeria, Babylon, Mesopotamia, and Assyria.

Middle Eastern cuisine has undergone thousands of years of refinement but has never lost touch with its roots. The home of many common herbs, the Middle East was also the source of sweet and sour sauces, stuffed grape leaves, pastries, and noodles. Some historians believe that pasta originated in Middle Eastern countries, most notably Libya, not in Italy. Worth emphasizing, too, is that yogurt is used widely in Middle Eastern cooking.

Here's how to adapt the 17 Day Diet to Middle Eastern dietary standards.

Cycle 1: Accelerate

Stick to the list of approved foods, but emphasize these cultural selections:

Cleansing vegetables

Asian eggplant

Zucchini

Grape leaves

Fruits

Persian lemon

Sour grapes

Cycle 2: Activate

Stick to the list of approved foods, but add these cultural selections:

Fruits

Barberries, popular in Middle Eastern cuisine for their slightly sour
flavor

Pomegranate

Cleansing Vegetables

Yellow peas

Probiotics

Labne, a thickened yogurt made by straining yogurt in cheese cloth
or a coffee filter overnight

Cycle 3: Achieve

Stick to the list of approved foods, but add these cultural selections:

Natural Starches

Thin flat bread (lavash)

General Tips

- Focus on traditional dishes that blend vinegar or lime juice with
vegetables. These lend themselves well to the 17 Day Diet. Another

is sabzi khordan, a plate of raw greens—green onions and watercress, mint and basil—which are eaten with your fingers, or tucked inside lavash with a slice of feta cheese.

- Make frittatas (kuku) with egg substitutes rather than eggs to cut calories and fat.

- Use brown rice instead of white rice in entrees.

- For probiotics, enjoy classic tzatziki, a yogurt cucumber dip made with garlic.

Now You're Cooking . . . and Losing Weight

The 17 Day Diet works for everyone, no matter what your culture or country of origin. The main reason is that it encompasses mostly natural foods, and these are found in all cuisines. I think you have to use some food commonsense, too: Inhaling too many greasy tacos, deep-fried egg rolls, or mountains of pasta will pack on pounds, mess with your cholesterol, clog your arteries, and, ultimately, set you up for heart disease.

Fortunately, following *The 17 Day Diet Breakthrough Edition* recommendations doesn't mean ditching your favorite recipes. Just use low-fat cooking techniques, concentrate on fruits and vegetables in their most natural state, and rely on probiotics like yogurt, which is a staple in many cultures. Be innovative, use some ingenuity, apply some creativity, and you will lose weight.

Review

- The 17 Day Diet is adaptable to any cuisine. One reason is that it emphasizes vegetables, fruits, lean protein, and whole grains—food groups that are a part of all cultures.

- Food preparation is key. Using less cooking fat and fewer starchy foods, you can make over many ethnic dishes to suit your diet.

- Be sensible: Eat smaller portions and avoid frying or otherwise cooking foods in too much fat.

- The 17 Day Diet is for everyone, no matter your cultural heritage or country of origin.

10

The PMS Exception Diet

There's always an exception to every rule, but most of the time I want you to follow them anyway. However, premenstrual syndrome (PMS) calls for bending the rules a bit.

Women, I'm sure you're happy and well-adjusted . . . until a few days before your period, when you turn into Attila the Hun and snap at everyone for no apparent reason. Your family and friends avoid you, and who would blame them?

Next come the physical symptoms, like your body being so bloated that it should be listed on MapQuest. Then, the cramps. On top of all this, it's hard to stay on your diet. When you're not doubled over with cramps, you're sticking your finger in a bottle of hot fudge sauce multiple times a day or eating more in one meal than Paris Hilton weighs.

Doctors still aren't sure why you get so out of sorts just prior to the arrival of your period, but we think it has to do with the ups and downs of estrogen and progesterone and how they lower the mood-lifting brain chemical serotonin. Serotonin is a chemical in your brain that, at proper levels, makes you feel happy. It's like a natural upper. When levels dip—which is what happens during PMS—you feel moody and crappy.

But here's what I want to emphasize: You don't have to be miserable during your time of the month. You can stick to a reasonable diet that one miserable week every month—and still lose weight. This is important, because being overweight or even obese makes PMS symptoms worse. You can accomplish this by following what I call the PMS Exception Diet. It's a combination of anti-PMS foods and supplements.

There are many lucky women who don't suffer from PMS and won't need this diet. The first step, before you consider this diet, is to determine: Do you suffer from PMS?

You might think that's a dumb question, and maybe it is. Most women know if they have PMS. Please humor me. Doctors went to school for eight years, and we like to put our medical training to use. We love asking questions to arrive at a diagnosis. Sometimes we even throw in a few unrelated questions, like "What kind of shampoo do you use?" or "Who played Carrie's California boyfriend on *Sex and the City?*"

Please take the following test. It will take just a second.

CHECK-UP: Do You Suffer from PMS?

Do you have any of these symptoms right before and/or during your period? Check off any of the symptoms that apply.

- ☐ Depression
- ☐ Headache
- ☐ Food cravings
- ☐ Bloat
- ☐ Cramps
- ☐ Feelings of sadness
- ☐ Desire to withdraw from social situations
- ☐ Irritability
- ☐ Fatigue
- ☐ Anxiety
- ☐ Nightmares
- ☐ Nausea
- ☐ Mood swings
- ☐ Breast tenderness
- ☐ Crying jags
- ☐ Sleep disturbances
- ☐ Hot flashes
- ☐ Weight gain

It's easier to diagnose a broken arm than premenstrual syndrome, but if you have five or more of these symptoms, then you're likely suffering from PMS. Fewer than five, and you've probably got simple menstrual discomfort.

MISTER M.D., CAN YOU PLEASE TELL ME

Aren't There Any Drugs My Doctor Can Prescribe for My PMS Symptoms?

Women have been suffering from PMS for years, and they are often treated with tranquilizers, antidepressants, and diuretics. Over-the-counter painkillers like ibuprofen are effective against cramps. But, honestly, simple changes in lifestyle (a healthy diet, exercise) have been found to be as effective as medication in relieving PMS troubles.

Diet and other lifestyle changes can help you beat PMS. I'll show you how to take charge right here. First, we'll look at foods that help ease symptoms; second, foods that aggravate symptoms and should be avoided; and third, how to modify the 17 Day Diet for one week to help you continue losing weight.

Eat to Beat PMS

I give my female patients lists of recommendations, and I help them decide what to incorporate. Of all the changes you can make to improve your premenstrual health, physicians and nutritional experts agree that adopting healthful eating habits will have the most immediate effect. Here is an overview of what to include on the PMS Exception Diet.

Salmon and Other Fish

For protein, fish like salmon, tuna, halibut, sardines, mackerel, and herring are excellent PMS-easing foods. The reason is, they're loaded with friendly omega-3 fatty acids. This friendly fat is a cramp reliever because it fights inflammation and pain. It also helps stabilize the hormonal swings that bring on so many PMS symptoms. So, if you're fishing for relief, catch some salmon!

One of the fatty acids in the omega-3s is DHA, short for *docosahexaenoic acid*. Low levels of DHA have been linked to depression. A study published in the medical journal *Lancet* stated that in regions where people ate more fish, there were fewer cases of depression. Another study, published in the *American Journal of Clinical Nutrition*, noted that the documented increase in depression in North America over the last century has paralleled the dwindling amount of DHA in our diets. Considering the evidence, I think it's a good idea to eat more fish. It seems to be a good natural treatment for depression.

Other nutrient gems from seafood include calcium, magnesium, iron, and zinc—all vital for easing symptoms.

One-Week PMS Exception Diet Prescription: Aim for at least 2 to 3 servings of seafood when experiencing symptoms.

Other Lean Proteins

Enjoying lean proteins such as lean meat and chicken helps you get *selenium*, an important anti-PMS mineral. Anxiety is associated with a deficiency in this mineral. Five weeks after psychologists at University College in Wales started administering a daily supplement of 100 micrograms of the mineral selenium to a group of 50 women and men, the subjects reported feeling more balanced and generally in better moods. Those who were low in selenium at the start reported the most dramatic mood boost. The U.S. Department of Agriculture has reported similar findings.

Other sources of selenium are seafood (particularly tuna) and whole grains. You can meet your entire daily selenium requirement by eating three Brazil nuts a day.

Include the following proteins this week:

Chicken breasts

Lean beef

Lean ground beef

3 Brazil nuts

One-Week PMS Exception Diet Prescription: Enjoy at least two servings of lean protein daily. Have 3 Brazil nuts every day during your period.

Soy Proteins

Tofu, tempeh, soy milk, and edamame (boiled, lightly salted soybeans in the pod) contain plant hormones called *isoflavones*, which may lessen PMS symptoms. There's evidence these natural compounds help your body absorb the extra estrogen and progesterone that play a role in making you feel moody, bloated, and crampy.

One-Week PMS Exception Diet Prescription: Enjoy soy foods as snacks a few times a week during your period.

Natural Carbohydrates

Carbohydrates are the dietary building blocks of serotonin, that wonderful feel-good chemical in your brain. Not all carbs are good at creating serotonin: I'm talking about simple carbs like sugar, sweets, and processed foods. In my practice, my women patients with PMS say their symptoms, particularly moodiness, are alleviated after they eat complex carbohydrates, such as whole grains, vegetables, and fruit. These foods are broken down more slowly by the body. This keeps blood sugar levels regulated, and serotonin, steady.

Carbs such as lima beans and black beans are high in potassium and magnesium—two minerals that help prevent mood swings, fatigue, cravings, and bloating. Sweet potatoes are rich in B vitamins, a family of nutrients that also help curb PMS symptoms.

One-Week PMS Exception Diet Prescription: Include 3 daily servings of the following:

½ cup cooked oatmeal

1 cup high-fiber cereal

1 slice whole-grain bread (no sugar added)

½ cup beans or legumes

1 medium sweet potato

½ cup corn

½ cup barley

½ cup brown rice

Water-Flushing Vegetables

A number of foods are thought to be *diuretics*, meaning that they help the body eliminate water. And most contain magnesium, potassium, calcium, and other nutrients that can relieve PMS. Asparagus, by the way, is one of the best. It contains a magical amino acid called *asparagine*. It works like a diuretic to flush excess fluids from your system. Vegetables are also full of fiber. It promotes regularity and, when you're regular, you don't bloat.

Eat the following vegetables during your period:

Asparagus

Beets

Cucumbers

Lettuce, all varieties

Parsley

Spinach

Tomatoes

Watercress

One-Week PMS Exception Diet Prescription: Eat water-flushing vegetables liberally each day.

Higher-Sugar Fruits

Like certain vegetables, many fruits are loaded with potassium, an anti-PMS nutrient. Some honorable mentions: banana, cantaloupe, grapes, and mangoes. Yes, these fruits are high in sugar, but that's a plus on this plan. Fruit is nature's candy and will help tame sugar cravings during your period.

Steer toward high-fiber fruits, too, such as apples, pears, and berries. Eat your fruit instead of drinking it, since fruit juice is almost pure sugar.

One-Week PMS Exception Diet Prescription: Enjoy up to 3 servings of fresh fruit daily, with an emphasis on the fruits discussed above.

Probiotics and Calcium Rich Foods

You're already eating probiotics on the 17 Day Diet. Well, guess what? These good bacteria can keep your system moving and free your body from bloat. In one study, women with abdominal pain, bloat, constipation, and/or diarrhea who took the probiotics in supplement form for four weeks noticed fewer of these annoying symptoms than those on a placebo.

Probiotic foods, such as yogurt, supply an important anti-PMS mineral: calcium. Research shows that women who take in 1,000 to 1,200 milligrams of calcium a day all month have fewer menstruation-related mood swings than do those who skimp on dairy products. When calcium is in short supply, hormone fluctuations worsen. Thus, getting enough of this mineral steadies your hormones and keeps serotonin on the upswing. You'll feel significantly less nervous, irritable, depressed, and moody.

One-Week PMS Exception Diet Prescription: Enjoy 2 servings of probiotics daily. Choose from the 17 Day Diet lists.

Anti-PMS Fats

Your body needs essential fatty acids (EFAs) to efficiently metabolize hormones. EFAs are a collection of polyunsaturated fats vital for bodily functions. *Essential* means that our body is unable to manufacture it, and we need to draw it daily from our diet.

To be of benefit to your body, EFAs are converted to prostaglandins. *Prostaglandins* are hormonelike substances responsible for the regulation of blood pressure, dilation of blood vessels for better circulation, prevention of clotting of the blood, reduction of inflammation, and regulation of insulin levels. They also act as a watchdog of the immune system.

Supplementation with EFAs that contain a fatty acid called *gamma-linolenic acid* (GLA) and/or omega-3 fats can help manage PMS symptoms. Evening primrose oil is high in GLA and is an effective anti-PMS supplement that can be taken in capsule form (see below). Flaxseed oil is loaded with omega-3s and is thus a great fat to eat during your period. It assists in hormonal regulation.

One-Week PMS Exception Diet Prescription: Have 1 to 2 tablespoons of flaxseed oil daily as your friendly fat serving. Talk to your doctor about taking supplemental fats.

Chocolate

The recommendation to eat a bit of chocolate during your period is controversial. Some docs say okay; others say no. I'm among those who believe that chocolate is an antidote for grumpiness. Everyone gets happy when they eat chocolate. It actually boosts the brain's production of serotonin, and chocolate contains *phenylethylamine*, the same brain chemical that gets jacked up when you're in love.

Chocolate has many other virtues. It's rich in magnesium, a calming mineral. If your love affair with chocolate is because of its nutritional qualities, go dark. Dark chocolate has the most cocoa content, and cocoa is the wonder substance. It's rich in *flavonoids*, a group of chemicals that protect the heart and blood vessels from tissue damage. (Milk chocolate is typically sweeter and less intense than dark chocolate, but much lower in flavonoids.)

So, go ahead, let chocolate make your day, but limit daily consumption to about ½ to 1 ounce of dark chocolate or some low-calorie cocoa. Of course, use moderation if you feel the urge—no eating both ears off a 6-foot chocolate bunny. Any benefit of chocolate will be wiped out if you gorge on it and gain weight. Don't deny your cravings during your period, but control them.

One-Week PMS Exception Diet Prescription: Enjoy ½ to 1 ounce of dark chocolate or some low-calorie cocoa during the week of your period, if you have a craving for chocolate.

Other Nutritional Tips to Fight PMS

Multiple meals. Aim to get five to six meals (breakfast, lunch, dinner, and snacks). The point is to maintain a steady blood-sugar level. A steady intake of foods high in complex carbs helps keep blood sugar high, so you're less affected by the hormone-induced irritability. Try not to go more than three hours without eating. Meals with a good balance of natural carbohydrates and a moderate amount of protein seem to do the trick for many women.

Water your body. One of the most annoying and frustrating symptoms of PMS is bloating. To fight it, drink plenty of water! This might seem counterintuitive, but as I've said, probably a zillion times, is to drink more water. That water will flush out excess fluids from your body. Unless you drink 8 to 10 cups of water daily, your body will think it's a dry well, and it will start hoarding water like crazy. That response will worsen your bloating.

MISTER M.D., CAN YOU PLEASE TELL ME

My Digestion Is So Out of Whack During My Period. What Can I Do?

What you're describing is fairly typical. Poor digestion can actually worsen PMS, so take the following precautions:

- Eat a variety of whole foods to ensure you get all the nutrients you need. Avoid canned, frozen, and otherwise processed foods.

- Eat freshly prepared foods whenever possible.

- Eat your heaviest meal around noon. The later in the day you eat, the lighter your meals should be. This helps with weight control, too.

- Chewing your food thoroughly makes it easier to digest.

- When preparing meals, create a peaceful, relaxed atmosphere in your kitchen to infuse your food with a healthful energy.

- If possible, eat at the same time every day.

- Eating warm or hot food promotes better digestion.

- Don't drink cold beverages; they decrease the digestive power in your stomach. Try drinking plain hot water flavored with freshly squeezed lemon juice.

What to Avoid

A number of foods and substances will make your symptoms worse. Avoid the following.

Soda. You don't drink this on the 17 Day Diet, and you definitely don't want to drink it during your period. The bubbles in carbonated drinks can make your belly bloat and protrude. Stick to plain water.

Gum. Chewing gum causes you to swallow excess air, which aggravates bloating. So when someone says you're full of hot air, you are. Spit your gum out.

PM Carbs. On the 17 Day Diet you don't eat carbs past 2:00 p.m. This is a good practice to follow during your period. Starchy foods like bread and pasta may cause you to retain water. Lay off them before bedtime to keep from waking up puffy.

Salt. Even a few shakes can be enough to promote bloating and breast tenderness. Cutting back on salt is a pretty easy change to make, and it can really help with your symptoms. Spice up foods with herbs, spices, low-sodium or no-salt seasonings, low-salt soy sauce, sea salt, or kelp.

Caffeine. I haven't told anyone about this but, one time, my nurses came into my office and caught me yelling at my pencil sharpener. They weren't alarmed, but gently said, "Dr. Moreno, we think you need to cut back on your coffee."

"What do you mean?" I wanted to know. "I can handle my coffee. It's not my fault that this pencil sharpener doesn't work."

They told me that I just seemed to be a little edgy lately. I was surprised. Like everyone else on earth, I drink a lot of coffee, a habit I picked up in med school to help me stay awake for 24 hours. I knew that coffee can increase irritability and mood swings. For women with PMS, coffee just aggravates all the emotional symptoms. In fact, studies confirm that the more coffee a woman drinks, the worse her PMS symptoms are. I don't have PMS, but I vowed to cut back on caffeine. Here's what I did. I did it gradually, no cold turkey, because that can bring on colossal headaches. Every couple of days, I trimmed my coffee intake by one-half cup. On days when I wanted a big mug of coffee, I cut my regular coffee with decaf. If you drink other sources of caffeine, such as teas and diet drinks, ease up on them too or switch to decaf versions.

Refined sugar. It's a no-no. White sugar hampers the absorption of magnesium, an important nutrient, and causes large fluctuations in blood-sugar levels, which can make you feel fatigued and robs your body of B vitamins. Stop stuffing yourself with sugar-laced comfort foods when you're feeling low. You'll feel much better if you steer clear of sweets. The immediate lift provided by sugar is usually followed by fatigue and, if you're already susceptible to depression, then being tired may make things look worse than ever.

Alcohol. Limit your intake to no more than one drink per day, or none at all, during your period. It can act as a depressant and make you irritable.

Eggs. During your period, pass up eggs in favor of egg whites. The fat content in eggs can interfere with the absorption of magnesium.

The PMS Exception Diet

Here's a look at an effective way to plan your meals during your period. Use these sample meals as a guideline to plan your own week of symptom-free living.

Day 1

Breakfast

- Cinnamon apple oatmeal: Peel and dice or grate 1 medium apple. Place the grated apple in a microwavable bowl with 2 to 3 tablespoons of water. Microwave on high for 3 minutes or until the apple is soft. Add the apple to a serving of cooked oatmeal. Serve and sprinkle with cinnamon. Cinnamon helps stabilize blood sugar.

Lunch

- Turkey sandwich: Two slices whole-grain bread, spread with a tablespoon of Dijon mustard, and slices of low-fat turkey breast and tomato slices
- 6 ounces fat-free plain or sugar-free yogurt with 1 cup diced mango

Dinner

- Grilled salmon
- Large salad of lettuce, tomatoes, and parsley, drizzled with 1 tablespoon of flaxseed oil and 2 tablespoons of herbed vinegar

Snacks

- 3 Brazil nuts
- 1 ounce dark chocolate
- 6 ounces plain low-fat or no-sugar-added yogurt, or 1 cup soy milk
- ½ medium cantaloupe

Day 2

Breakfast

- Cheesy parfait: Combine ½ cup Breakstone LiveActive cottage cheese with 1 cup berries (any variety) and 3 chopped Brazil nuts

Lunch

- 1½ cups whole-wheat pasta (this constitutes your 3 servings of natural carbs for the day) topped with sugar-free marinara sauce
- 1 medium apple or pear

Dinner

- Grilled or baked chicken
- Plenty of steamed asparagus
- Sliced tomato, drizzled with 1 tablespoon flaxseed oil and herbs
- ½ cup low-fat chocolate pudding

Snacks

- 6 ounces fat-free plain or sugar-free yogurt
- 1 medium banana

Day 3

Breakfast

- 1 cup cocoa made with soy milk
- 2 scrambled egg whites
- 1 slice whole-grain toast
- ½ medium cantaloupe

Lunch

- Tuna sandwich: Mix a 3 oz. can of tuna with a tablespoon of light mayonnaise and 3 tablespoons finely diced celery. Serve on whole-grain bread with tomato slices.
- 6 ounces fat-free plain or no-sugar-added yogurt with 1 cup diced mango

Dinner

- Grilled steak
- Large salad of lettuce, tomatoes, and parsley drizzled with 1 tablespoon flaxseed oil and 2 tablespoons herbed vinegar

Snacks

- 1 medium apple or pear
- 3 Brazil nuts
- Large bowl edamame

Day 4

Breakfast

- 1 cup high-fiber cereal
- 1 medium banana, sliced, added to cereal
- 1 cup soy milk

Lunch

- Large spinach salad with spinach leaves, topped with ½ cup of tofu (cubed), 2 slices cooked turkey bacon (crumbled), ½ cup garbanzo beans, and chopped parsley, drizzled with fat-free dressing
- 1 slice whole-grain bread
- 6 ounces fat-free plain or no-sugar-added yogurt with 1 cup fresh berries

Dinner

- Grilled pork chops
- Cucumber and tomato salad. Slice half a cucumber, combine with 1 cup of grape tomatoes, and drizzle with 1 tablespoon flaxseed oil and 2 tablespoons herbed vinegar.

Snacks

- 3 Brazil nuts
- 1 ounce dark chocolate
- 6 ounces fat-free plain or no-sugar-added yogurt
- 1 medium apple or pear

Day 5

Breakfast

- Cheese toast: Top 2 slices whole-grain bread with 3 tablespoons shredded reduced-fat cheddar cheese. Broil until cheese melts.
- 1 cup melon balls

Lunch

- Chef's salad: Large bed of lettuce, chopped cucumber, ½ cup garbanzo beans, sliced pickled beets, and strips of baked chicken or turkey drizzled with 1 tablespoon flaxseed oil and 2 tablespoons herbed vinegar.
- 6 ounces fat-free plain or sugar-free yogurt with 1 cup fresh berries

Dinner

- Grilled or baked salmon
- Steamed asparagus
- ½ cup low-fat chocolate pudding

Snacks

- 1 cup fresh pineapple chunks
- 3 Brazil nuts
- Large bowl edamame

Day 6

Breakfast

- Smoothie: In a blender, combine ½ cup soy milk, 6 ounces light or fat-free plain yogurt, 1 sliced banana, a dash of vanilla extract, and 4 ice cubes.
- 1 slice whole-grain toast

Lunch

- Boiled or steamed shrimp
- ½ cup lima beans

- ½ cup corn
- 1 medium apple or pear

Dinner

- Grilled steak
- Mixed green salad with parsley, chopped cucumbers, and grape tomatoes, drizzled with 1 tablespoon flaxseed oil and 2 tablespoons seasoned or balsamic vinegar
- One 5-ounce glass of red wine

Snacks

- 3 Brazil nuts
- 1 ounce dark chocolate
- 6 ounces fat-free plain or no-sugar-added yogurt
- ½ medium cantaloupe or 1 cup strawberries

Day 7

Breakfast

- 2 scrambled egg whites
- ½ cup oatmeal
- 1 cup berries

Lunch

- Lean hamburger patty
- 1 cup brown rice
- Stewed tomatoes
- 6 ounces fat-free plain or no-sugar-added yogurt
- 1 medium apple or pear

Dinner

- Roasted turkey breast
- Steamed asparagus

- Cucumber and tomato salad: Slice half a cucumber, combine with a cup of grape tomatoes, and drizzle with 1 tablespoon flaxseed oil and 2 tablespoons seasoned vinegar
- One 5 ounce glass of red wine

Snacks

- 3 Brazil nuts
- 1 ounce dark chocolate
- 6 ounces fat-free plain or no-sugar-added yogurt
- 1 medium banana

LEAN 17: 17 Bloat Busters

It's Saturday night, and you slip on your sexiest black dress. One problem: Your stomach is so swollen that the dress barely zips and your tummy is pooching out. Sound familiar? Bloating is a common but annoying PMS symptom with many causes. It's usually due to the hormonal changes that happen right before your period arrives. Luckily, there are easy ways to banish bloat, 17 in all.

Supplement Savvy for PMS

The pills I do like to throw at medical problems are nutritional supplements. There are many supplements you can take on a regular basis that can help. Consult your doctor about considering the following:

Multivitamin/mineral. Take one in the morning with food. (If taking children's vitamins, take 2 tablets.) Taking a multi with food optimizes the absorption of the vitamins and minerals, especially B6, magnesium, and potassium—nutrients that help ease premenstrual distress. Vitamin B6 is important for helping the liver regulate excess estrogen levels and has been shown to help prevent menstrual cramps.

Vitamin D. Sufficient daily intake of vitamin D (400 IU) may alleviate PMS symptoms, particularly irritability.

Calcium carbonate. At least 1,200 milligrams. On average, your diet probably provides only 600 to 800 milligrams of calcium a day, not the 1,000 to 1,200 mg necessary to ease your PMS symptoms. One study found that women who took this much calcium cut the severity of their PMS symptoms in half. Calcium appears to enhance the brain's processing of serotonin.

Magnesium. 400 milligrams twice daily. This mineral has a calming effect. It is also good for digestion. Whole grains and lentils are loaded with it, but you can also get it in a multiple vitamin-mineral supplement. Magnesium improves mood, and one study has shown it can provide significant relief if you suffer from menstrual headaches. Magnesium citrate, aspartate, and glycinate are better absorbed than the oxide form.

Fish oil. Three grams daily. Up your dosage to 5 grams daily when PMS symptoms begin.

Evening primrose oil. 1,000 milligrams daily. It relieves one of the most common PMS symptoms: breast tenderness.

1. Stop eating high-sodium stuff like canned soups, fast food, and cured meats. Sodium causes your body to hang on to water.

2. Drink more water. Believe it or not, extra fluids will help to flush out the sodium—and the bloat.

3. Avoid simple carbs (think white bread, white pasta, chips, etc.). Carbs get broken down into glucose and stored in the body as glycogen for energy. In order to be stored, a water molecule must attach to that glucose. The more stored carbs you have, the heavier you'll feel.

4. Opt for high-fiber carbs like vegetables and fruit. The longer food sits in your intestines, the more likely you are to retain water.

5. Exercise. It sweats out excess water and speeds up digestion. When you exercise, you stimulate the muscles that help move food and water through your system faster. Fight constipation by walking for at least 17 minutes each day to keep food moving through your digestive tract. Working up a sweat also releases fluids. In addition, research shows that moderate exercise soothes cramps, headaches, and lower-back pain; improves sleep; and reduces fatigue. And exercise boosts endorphin levels, which helps improve your mood.

6. Take calcium and magnesium, as I mentioned. Both compete with sodium for absorption into your body, so if you take in adequate amounts of either, your body is forced to flush out the salt that wasn't effectively absorbed.

7. Be wary of diuretics. When you stop taking a diuretic, your body retains more water, making you bloat for one to two weeks afterward. This can lead to a physical dependency so that your body needs the drug to rid itself of the excess fluid instead of doing it naturally.

8. Shun sodas. I just cannot overstate this recommendation. The caffeine in sodas dehydrates you, and phosphorous, a common soda additive, can inflame your intestinal wall, making you feel even puffier.

9. Discuss the appropriateness of birth control pills with your physician. Birth control pills may stabilize your level of progesterone, a bloat-inducing hormone.

10. Boost your B6. Many PMS symptoms, including water retention, are triggered by a defect in your body's metabolism of vitamin B6. Take 50 to 100 milligrams of B6 daily to see if it helps.

11. Stop the junk. Reduce your intake of foods that are difficult to digest, such as sugary, fatty, and fried fare, which can sit in your gut, causing constipation and distention.

12. Enjoy water-flushing vegetables.

13. To beat bloat, try a natural diuretic drink, such as a cup of chamomile or dandelion tea, or a glass of noncarbonated water with lemon or lime.

14. The artificial sweetener sorbitol, found in some sugarless gums and candies, can contribute to bloating, as can the consumption of alcohol, caffeine, and even nicotine.

15. Also avoid dairy products that contain lactose—milk sugar—if they seem to worsen your bloating symptoms.

16. Up your protein the week before and during your period. Protein has a diuretic effect on the body.

17. Take supplemental probiotics.

If the changes I'm recommending seem too daunting, try making just a few at a time. My patients tell me that eating more regularly, eliminating refined sugar and caffeine, plus exercising more, make the biggest difference. Or target your most bothersome symptoms: If your breasts really bother you, for example, try taking evening primrose oil or cutting out salt to see if you get relief.

To assess whether the PMS Exception Diet is working for you, you really have to try it for at least 6 cycles. Keep track of how your body reacts. As your symptoms decrease, I think you'll be motivated to stick to this diet. If an annoying symptom persists, or you keep gaining weight, consult your doctor. Keep in mind your ultimate objectives: relief of PMS symptoms and ongoing weight loss.

Review

- Several minor adjustments in the 17 Day Diet can help you during your period. Include more omega-3 rich foods such as salmon, increase your daily intake of natural carbs to 3 servings a day, eat more water-flushing vegetables, and enjoy higher-sugar fruits.
- Probiotics and calcium-rich foods help with digestion problems and mood swings.
- Eat a bit of chocolate during your period. It helps with stress relief.
- Eat multiple meals (5 to 6 daily) to maintain a steady blood-sugar level.
- Avoid soda, chewing gum, p.m. carbs, too much salt or caffeine, refined sugar, and eggs.
- Several supplements can help: a multivitamin/mineral; vitamin D, calcium, magnesium, fish oil, and evening primrose oil.
- Employ bloat-busting strategies, including drinking lots of water throughout the day.

THE 17 MINUTE WORKOUT: Sunlight Soothes PMS Symptoms

Outdoor aerobic activity is best if you're trying to alleviate PMS discomfort. Sunlight has been shown to reverse depression, carbohydrate cravings, fatigue, and irritability in women with PMS. Spending too much time indoors under artificial light can make PMS symptoms worse.

So, try some brisk walking, playing tennis, running, hiking, or biking. These are all activities that contribute to a heightened sense of relaxation and well-being. Aerobic exercise, in general, elevates the production of *endorphins*—brain chemicals that have a soothing effect. It also helps keep your heart and bones healthy and relieves muscle tension.

In addition to regular aerobic activity, the next best exercise prescription for PMS includes yoga to stretch muscles, align the spine, and increase mental focus. However, don't overdo exercise, since excessive exercise causes irregular periods or the cessation of menstruation and unhealthful conditions that can lead to the premature loss of bone.

PART FOUR

....

Make It Stick

11

Dining Out on the 17 Day Diet

N o one is at home anymore. Where are we? We're sitting in restaurants. On average, Americans dine out four times a week, according to the National Restaurant Association. And now habitual restaurant eating has been linked to the rise in obesity, because restaurants serve gigantic portions, filled with hidden fats and sugars. Statisticians calculate that each person in the U.S. spends $1,117 a year dining out, and I know people who spend that much in a month! Our wallets are getting slimmer but not our waistlines. Yikes! I guess you have to ask yourself if you want to be overweight or rich.

When we dine out, most of our meals don't even include a cloth napkin because we're eating at fast food joints. Fast food restaurants are everywhere, even in hospitals. That means you can get your high-fat, high-calorie fast food and your medical care in the same place. Unfortunately, your insurance company does not reimburse you for these meals.

Hospitals claim these restaurants are not for patients, but for the visitors and employees. Sure. Anyone who works in a hospital knows that a lot of that food will be smuggled into patients' rooms. When you're sick in bed in the hospital, you know who your true friends are and they're not bringing flowers and balloons.

Hospitals have gotten savvy in other ways. Did you know some even offer room service? That's right. Meals are served bedside by waiters in black tie and crisp burgundy jackets. This makes you feel like you're in a restaurant, only you're lying on your back in a hospital gown, staring up at the ceiling, and developing a new appreciation for acoustic tile.

"Hi, my name is Walter, and I'll be your waiter."

Just when you think you get to place an order for filet mignon, garlic mashed potatoes, and cheesecake, Walter says: "Would you like red, green, or yellow Jell-O with your meatloaf?" Your heart sinks and you reluctantly say, "Red Jell-O."

Regardless of where you eat out (hospitals or otherwise), you might be surprised to see just how high the calorie counts of some restaurant meals are. A healthy-sounding chicken fajita omelet at IHOP, for instance, weighs in at 1,360 calories. If you think about the fact that the recommended daily calorie intake for adults runs from 1,600 to 2,800 calories a day, eating that omelet takes a huge bite out of your recommended calorie intake.

Think you're making a healthy choice if you order carrot cake at the Cheesecake Factory? Not so fast. According to the restaurant's materials in 2013, one slice of carrot cake slice gives you 1,550 calories. Consider a Taco Bell Fiesta Taco Salad with Beef: 780 calories and 42 grams of fat. That hurts! Or a medium-size Starbucks Caffe Mocha eaten with a Blueberry Scone has a whopping 720 calories and 46 grams of fat.

These numbers are no big secrets. They are posted on restaurants' websites, and often on menus. Pay attention to them; they can help you make healthy, informed choices.

If you chowed down on this stuff, unrestrained, you've just booked yourself a trip to Obesity Land and Disease City. I'm not going to say don't eat out. I'm going to talk to you about eating healthy when you eat out. You can dine out successfully on the 17 Day Diet and enjoy your experience by learning how to navigate any menu. These days, more restaurants than ever offer low-fat, low-cal menu items, making it easy to enjoy a delicious, nutritious dining experience, if you know what to ask for. Let me offer some tips that will help you eat smart while dining out.

LEAN 17: The 17 Most Fattening Restaurant Choices

Menu Item	Calories*
1. Fried seafood combo platter (with 4 tbsp. tartar sauce, fries, coleslaw, and 2 biscuits with 2 pats of butter)	2,170
2. Fried chicken dinner, with a biscuit and mashed potatoes	2,000
3. Cheese fries (1 order with ranch dressing)	1,980
4. General Tso's Chicken with rice	1,600
5. Bloomin Onion	1,959
6. Molten chocolate cake with ice cream	1,270
7. Fettuccine Alfredo	1,220
8. Stuffed potato skins (8 skins with 5 tbsp. sour cream)	1,140
9. Ribeye (14 ounces)	1,055

*Calorie counts at particular restaurants may vary.

10.	Fried calamari	1,000
11.	Cheese quesadilla or chicken burrito	1,000
12.	Fast food shake, large	980
13.	Cheesecake (⅙ of the cake)	970
14.	Spaghetti with meatballs	920
15.	Kung Pao chicken with rice	900
16.	Combo Lo mein noodle dish	710
17.	Beef and broccoli with rice	710

Know Before You Go

With most restaurants these days, you can go online and look at their menus. See what dishes look healthy—grilled items, salads, vegetable sides, and so forth. Decide before you go what you'll order, and stick to your decision once you get there. Collect the menus in the restaurants you frequent so that you have them to refer to.

Sit in a Quiet Spot

Nobody knows this, but people who sit in the noisiest sections of restaurants (by large parties of partiers or lots of kids, by a window, or in front of a television) chow down more than those in quieter areas. A lot of noise, activity, and commotion distract us from how much we eat. I always ask for the quietest corner of the restaurant because I like to relax while I enjoy my meal, and I do this when I make my reservation, just to be on the safe side. If it's an establishment that doesn't take reservations, ask for a quiet spot when you get there.

Be the First to Order

Here's where you really need to take charge. If you're watching your weight and want to eat out lean, dispense briefly with good manners and order first. If you don't, you might be tempted by your friend's order of something decadent like Fettuccine Alfredo and begin to rethink your boring grilled chicken. If you still want to be polite, look at the menu, make your decision, close your menu, and stick to your choice. Also, maybe your non-dieting friend will take a cue from you and order something healthy. Congratulate yourself for sticking to your food guns and setting a good example.

Have It Your Way

Before ordering your selections, ask the server about the details of the meal. This will help you make more informed choices. Some questions to ask include:

- How is this dish prepared? Can it be modified?
- What ingredients are used?
- Do you have any low-fat or low-calorie options?
- What comes with this meal?
- Can I make substitutions?
- How large are the portions?

Don't be afraid to make special requests. For example, ask that foods be served with minimal butter, margarine, or oil. Ask if a particular dish can be broiled or baked rather than fried. Also, ask that no additional salt be added to your food.

You may also be able to make substitutions. If the ingredients are on the menu, the chef should be able to accommodate your needs. A common substitution is a baked potato for fries, or a double serving of vegetables instead of a starch. If your dish does not arrive at the table the way you ordered it, don't be afraid to send it back.

If you don't see something you like, ask for it. As a paying customer, you have the right to eat not only what tastes good, but what's good for you. Be weight assertive!

ROBERTA: I Broke Through!

I am a 43-year-old mother of two. Over the years, my metabolism had slowed down and, in combination with a lack of exercise and poor diet, I found myself overweight and unhappy. A co-worker mentioned *The 17 Day Diet* book that she was reading and how it had worked for a few of her friends. I immediately went out and purchased it. My life hasn't been the same since!

My starting weight was 211 pounds. When I first started the 17 Day Diet program, I couldn't keep the weight on if I tried. Every day that I stepped on the scale, I was down in weight and my clothes were fitting a lot looser. By the end of the program, I weighed 156 pounds—a loss of 55 pounds. I went from a size 16 to a size 8.

The book was so helpful, as it not only gave me the knowledge as to what types of foods I can and should be eating, or how to avoid making bad food choices at parties or when eating out, it also included recipes! For someone who would walk into the grocery store and completely pass by the fresh vegetables with no clue what to buy or how to cook them, I was so excited to have a guide and suggestions as to the different types of foods I should be eating. I now crave vegetables and confidently load up my cart with healthy and nutritious foods.

It may have initially started out being called a diet, but very soon after I realized that it really was a lifestyle change. We should all be aware of the foods we have been eating and the damage it is doing to our bodies. Not only have I become a healthier person, I have also passed on healthy eating habits to my children.

I recall that, in the first 6 months or so of starting this new healthy way of living, often wondering if I was just dreaming that I was a thinner and happier person. It has been almost two years since I started that program, and life couldn't be better for me now. I have been successful at maintaining my weight. I no longer have knee and ankle pain, stomach aches and headaches. I live an active lifestyle by walking or biking daily. I feel alive and healthy!

Thank you, Dr. Moreno, for this book. I truly believe it has saved my life.

Before   *After*

Don't Be Seduced by Menu Descriptions

You open the menu and there are pictures: stacks of pancakes with sugary fillings, skyscraper-high burgers overfilling with cheese and bacon, or ribs dripping in mouth-watering sauce. If there are no photos, the descriptions of each menu item tease and taunt you: "tender, juicy chicken breasts," "knife-tender prime rib," or "classic lasagna." These photos and words are meant to seduce you; there's no question about it. And it works. Studies reveal that descriptions promoting the delectable attributes of menu items can increase a restaurant's sales by 23 percent, and can even influence how the food tastes to you! They prime your sense of taste and smell to expect something delicious. Ah, the power of advertising!

Here's what I do to prevent from being put under the spell of restaurant advertising. I make a game out of picking the descriptive, alluring adjectives on the menu. We see who can find the most in three minutes. If I win, everyone buys me dinner. That's the rule of the game.

Stay Away from Snacking

I rarely order appetizers, because I am guaranteed to spoil my main meal. Appetizers take away your appetite for the healthiest foods to come. Avoid them. Even the freebies like chips and salsa at Mexican restaurants, or a basket of rolls and butter at other establishments, can pile up fat and calories that you don't need. If you can't exercise control, have your server remove the temptation.

Make a Meal out of Appetizers

Certain appetizers can be excellent choices for an entrée. The portion size of appetizers is often more appropriate than the extremely large portions provided in entrées. Consider healthful options such as steamed or poached seafood (for example, shrimp cocktail), salads that aren't loaded with high-fat ingredients (such as cheese and bacon), grilled vegetables, and broth-based soups. You might also choose to combine the appetizer with a salad; the salad will bulk up the meal so that you feel more satisfied without adding a lot of calories. Be aware that some appetizers, particularly fried fare or items covered in cheeses, oils, and cream sauces, may be overloaded with calories and fat. Some fried appetizers can provide a day's worth of fat for four people!

Be Salad Savvy

Salad lovers, beware! A salad can be the healthiest item at a restaurant, or the most fattening, if you drown it in high-fat dressings, croutons, cheese, or bacon. The best move is to have a salad made with fresh greens and veggies, served with vinaigrette, low-cal dressing, even a generous squeeze of fresh lemon.

One of the best ways to manage the fat and calories is to order the dressing on the side and use the fork-dip method to eat your salad. (You won't look funny doing this, because everyone who has ever been on a diet knows how to do the fork-dip method.) Dip the tines of your salad fork in the dressing, then spear the leaves of your salad. That way, you get a taste of the dressing with each bite of salad.

If you want to be really good, carry one of those salad spritzer products in your purse. Order your salad without dressing. Pull out your spritzer and spray your salad. Be aware, though, that this might scare the other patrons, who will think you are sanitizing your salad.

And watch out for potato salads, macaroni salads, coleslaw, and even tuna and chicken salads, which usually are heavy in mayonnaise, sugar, and calories.

Go Low on Sides

Depending on the cycle you're on, substitute high-cal side dishes with low-fat options such as steamed vegetables, brown rice, or fresh fruit. Forget the French fries, and have baked, boiled, or roasted potatoes, leaving off the butter, cheese, and creams. Flavor with salsa or pepper and chives instead.

Choose Low-Fat Preparation Methods

The way your entrée is prepared affects its calorie and fat content. Choose grilled, broiled, or baked meats and entrees. Pan-fried and deep-fried foods give you extra fat you don't need. I can't say this in too many ways or too many times, but broiling, baking, steaming, poaching, and grilling sea-food, skinless poultry, lean meat, and veggies give you all the flavor with-out all the fat.

For example, grilled chicken is lower in fat and calories than fried chicken. (If you are served chicken with skin, you can remove the skin to save significant fat and calories.)

It's not easy to get rid of all fat in restaurant meals, but give it a try. Ask the server if the butter or oil used to prepare your entrée can be reduced or eliminated. Even a grilled item may have extra fat added. For example, some grilled beef dishes call for added oil.

Drink Water with Your Meal

Here is one of my favorite tips: Drink all of the water served to you at a res-taurant, and when the first glass runs out, have the server refill your glass. Sometimes I watch how much water my dinner companions drink at a meal. If they have barely touched their water glass, I point it out to them and talk about how important it is to stay hydrated. Hey, I am a doctor. I don't always leave everything at the office.

Water will prevent you from drinking too much alcohol, it will fill you up so that you don't overeat, and it will help your body flush out fatten-ing stuff and other hidden gook from the restaurant meal. Besides, water at restaurants somehow tastes better than a glass of water from home. I am not a water snob; I just like the taste of restaurant water!

Enjoy Alcohol in Moderation

Drinks can be diet busters, too. Ice water is free, but fancy mixed drinks have lots of empty calories, and the alcohol can dull your reasoning and inhibitions. Because alcohol can contribute significant amounts of calo-ries, limiting your intake to 150 calories' worth is a good idea. The follow-ing portions of alcohol each contain 150 calories or less: 5 ounces of wine, 1.5 ounces of liquor, or 12 ounces of light beer.

Many people find it helpful to order wine by the glass rather than the bottle, so that they can better control and monitor their intake. You can decide ahead of time at which point in the meal your beverage would be most satisfying. For example, you may want to save your glass of wine for your entrée and sip water while you wait for your meal. Holding off on alcohol until a later course also helps to decrease alcohol's effect on your inhibitions. If you drink alcohol on an empty stomach, it can relax you to the point that you lose sight of your game plan. Setting a personal limit and planning when to enjoy your beverage should help you stick with your goals.

Practice Portion Control

Restaurants serve mountains of food—about two to three times the quantity that we need in a meal. This is no big secret. Just don't try to finish those megasized portions. Consider sharing a meal or taking a doggie bag so that you can have a quick meal at a later time. Eat until you're satisfied, not stuffed, and take the rest home. As you're eating, use my Hunger/ Fullness Meter, listen to your internal hunger signals, and stop when you have had enough. Eating slowly helps you recognize such cues.

Keep track of how much you eat, and stick to the number of servings you planned to eat. You probably won't bring a scale with you to the restaurant so that you can measure out portions, but you can rely on visual references. For example:

- A serving of cooked meat, chicken, or fish is like the palm of your hand, or about the size of a deck of cards.
- A serving of green salad is like an open-palmed hand.
- A serving of fruit or vegetable is like your fist, or about the size of a tennis ball.
- A serving of baked potato is the size of a baseball.
- An ounce of cheese is like your pointer and index fingers together, or about the size of four stacked dice.
- A serving of salad dressing is like your thumb.
- A 3-ounce hamburger patty is the size of a quart-size mayonnaise jar lid.

Practice the Three-Bite Rule

Try to satisfy your sweet tooth with fresh fruit, and that's it. Wave off the dessert cart. Don't even order dessert, unless you're on Cycle 4 and are enjoying weekends off.

That said, you can also practice my three-bite rule with dessert, if you want to watch your calories a little more strictly.

There are lots of variations on the three-bite rule, by the way. Moms try the three-bite rule all the time. "Johnny, you must eat at least three bites of everything on your plate before you're excused from the table." This usually does not work. Mothers spend many long, painful, tearful hours in a standoff, while kids discover at least 152 ways to say *disgusting*.

My variation on the three-bite rule is different. If you truly want molten chocolate lava cake, go ahead and order it, but just have a taste. Take three bites and then set it aside for a few minutes, or let your dinner companions have some. You're less likely to come back to it. There is no way you can gain weight with three bites of anything.

Incidentally, servers use the three-bite rule all the time. After they serve the food, they wait until you have had three bites. Then they come back and ask if everything is okay.

If you're being good on your diet, you will ask the server to remove the rest of the dessert. Be careful here. This may hurt the chef's feelings. You have to soften the blow by explaining to your server that you, too, are practicing the three-bite rule.

Choose Wisely at Any Meal

Looking for more healthy ideas while dining out? These general suggestions can help you make good choices at almost any restaurant.

Breakfast

Cereal with skim milk topped with fruit

Oatmeal with fruit or raisins and skim milk

Wheat, rye, or whole-grain toast

Eggs, egg substitutes, or egg whites (including omelets)

Low-fat or light yogurt

Fresh fruit

Appetizers

Gazpacho or vegetable juice

Broth, bouillon, or consommé

Vegetable soup without cream

Shrimp cocktail

Steamed clams or mussels

Green salad, without meat or cheese, with dressing on the side

Vegetable antipasto

Vegetables

Steamed, stewed, boiled, or grilled vegetables without butter or sauces

Starches

Baked or boiled potatoes, no butter

Baked sweet potato, no butter

Pasta or steamed rice (whole-wheat pasta and brown rice are preferable)

Entrees

Lean meats: grilled, broiled, or served au jus (trimmed of excess fat)

Fish or skinless poultry: grilled, steamed, baked, broiled, or poached
in wine, lemon juice, or lime juice (without added fat)

Ahi tuna

Beverages

Water, mineral water, seltzer, tea, or coffee (unsweetened)

Virgin Bloody Mary

Glass of dry red or white wine

Fast Food Choices

Grilled chicken, hold the bun

Entree salads

Movie Snacks

Kid-sized box of popcorn

Bottle of water

Dill pickle (Yes, many movie theaters serve these. But be careful
when you bite down or else you will spray pickle juice on the
head of the guy in front of you and create a commotion.)

Here are some other ways to choose wisely at just about any restaurant.

Best Choices at Ethnic Restaurants	
Asian	• Steamed rice • Steamed Chinese vegetables • Stir-fry vegetables with shrimp/chicken • Teriyaki beef or chicken • Steamed or baked tofu (make sure it is not fried) and vegetables • Hot-and-sour soup • Miso soup • Entrees made with chicken or fish and vegetables • Steamed chicken and vegetables with a half cup of brown rice • Any boiled, steamed, or lightly stir-fried seafood, chicken, vegetable, or tofu dishes • Sushi • Sashimi • Edamame
Delicatessen	• Half a deli sandwich—roast turkey with mustard on rye • Lox with tomato and onion • Low-fat deli meats, such as low-fat turkey or even low-fat ham • Salad with dressing on the side • Whole-wheat bread, rye, or pumpernickel

French	• Poached fish entrees
	• Roasted or grilled lean meats
	• Bouillabaisse
	• Salade Nicoise
	• Broth-based soups
	• Plain vegetables
Greek/Middle Eastern	• Yogurt-based dips
	• Meat and vegetables on a skewer
	• Grilled meat entrees
	• Stuffed pepper with meat and rice
	• Cabbage rolls
	• Tabouli
	• Vegetable dishes and soups
Indian	• Any dish with beans, rice, grains, vegetables
	• Chicken tandoori
	• Vegetable curry
	• Shrimp bhuna
	• Fish vindaloo
	• Lentil soup
	• Salad or vegetables with yogurt dressing
Italian	• Minestrone
	• Vegetable antipasto
	• Mussels with marinara sauce
	• Chicken Marsala
	• Clams with marinara sauce
	• Spaghetti squash with marinara (some Italian restaurants have this variety of squash on their menus; it makes a delicious, low-calorie substitute for pasta)
	• Chicken cacciatore
	• Veal piccata
	• Grilled chicken or fish entrees

Mexican	• Grilled foods such as chicken or fish
	• Salsa
	• Pico de gallo
	• Tortilla soup
	• Black or red beans
	• Black bean soup
	• Mexican rice
	• Chili with beans
	• Salad, dressing on the side

Stay healthy but leave room to be flexible when you eat out: Eating is an integral—and fun—part of life, and life can be unpredictable. An unexpected change in your daily eating plan isn't the end of the world. In fact, you can enjoy dining out even more if you remember that it's your total diet that counts, not individual meals. You're always going to eat out at restaurants. Hopefully, you'll eat a little differently most of the time.

Review

- Be prepared before you go out to eat at a restaurant. Check out online menus and decide what you will order.

- Sit in a quiet spot (people eat more in noisy restaurants) and be the first to order, so that you're not influenced by what your friends order.

- Stand your ground with the waitstaff. Remember, you are a paying customer. Ask how foods are prepared, and request that your order be prepared according to healthy cooking methods.

- Make an appetizer your main meal, since appetizer portions are often smaller than meal entrees.

- Order salad dressing on the side.

- Don't try to drink and diet; too much alcohol can make you ravenous and make you forget that you're dieting.

- Practice portion control. Don't eat everything on your plate; take some home for lunch or dinner the next day.

- Try the three-bite rule, especially for desserts.

CHECK-UP: Dr. Mike's Restaurant Quiz—How Much Do You Know about Nutrition at Popular Restaurants?

If you're trying to reduce the calories and fat in your diet, dining out can be a challenge. Take my quiz to test your restaurant smarts.

1. Which 6-inch sandwich at Subway has the fewest calories?

   A. Subway Club

   B. Tuna Salad

   C. Roast Beef

   D. Steak and Cheese

2. Which breakfast item at McDonald's has the most calories?

   A. Steak, Egg, and Cheese Bagel

   B. Hotcakes with syrup

   C. Egg McMuffin

   D. Sausage Burrito

3. Which salad at Subway has the most calories?

   A. Black Forest Ham Salad

   B. Turkey Breast Salad

   C. Sweet Onion Chicken Teriyaki Salad

   D. Veggie Delite Salad

4. Which of the following from TCBY has the fewest calories?

   A. ½ cup no-sugar-added vanilla frozen yogurt

   B. ½ cup orange sorbet

5. Of the types of pizza you can order at Pizza Hut, which variety has the most calories (based on ⅛ medium 12-inch pizza)?

   A. Cheese Pan Pizza

   B. Medium Cheese Thin 'N Crispy Pizza

   C. Hand Tossed Cheese Pizza

   D. Veggie Lover's Pan Pizza

6. What is the average calorie count of a 20-ounce Slim N Trim smoothie at Smoothie King?

   A. 362 calories

   B. 283 calories

   C. 422 calories

   D. 195 calories

7. Which muffin at Dunkin' Donuts has the most calories?

   A. Corn Muffin

   B. Coffee Cake Muffin

   C. Blueberry Muffin

   D. Honey Bran Raisin Muffin

8. What is the lowest-calorie plate you can order at Boston Market?

   A. Turkey Breast (regular)

   B. Beef Brisket (regular)

   C. Half Rotisserie Chicken

   D. Pastry Top Turkey Pot Pie

9. What is the average calorie count of a seafood entree at Captain D's Seafood?

   A. 224

   B. 758

   C. 589

   D. 350

10. Which 16-ounce drink at Starbucks has the most calories?

   A. Hot Chocolate

   B. Flavored Latte

   C. Cappuccino

   D. Caffe Mocha

How did you do? The answers may surprise you:

1. The correct answer is A (Subway Club) at 310 calories. The Roast Beef sandwich weighs in at 320 calories; the Steak and Cheese sandwich, 380 calories; and the Tuna Salad sandwich, 480 calories.

2. The correct answer is A (Steak, Egg, and Cheese Bagel). It has 630 calories. Hot Cakes have 350 calories. The Egg McMuffin and the Sausage Burrito have 300 calories each.

3. The correct answer is C (Sweet Onion Chicken Teriyaki Salad) at 240 calories. The Black Forest Ham Salad and the Turkey Breast Salad have 110 calories each. The Veggie Delite Salad contains 60 calories.

4. The correct answer is A (½ cup no-sugar-added vanilla frozen yogurt) at 80 calories. The ½ cup of orange sorbet contains 100 calories.

5. The correct answer is D (a slice of Veggie Lover's Pan Pizza) at 107 calories. The slice of Medium Thin 'N Crispy Cheese Pizza has 65 calories; the slice of Hand Tossed Cheese Pizza, 84 calories; and the Cheese Pan Pizza, 91 calories.

6. The correct answer is B (283 calories). The lowest calorie smoothie in the Slim N Trim category is Orange Vanilla at 208 calories; the highest calorie smoothie in that category is Strawberry.

7. The correct answer is B (Coffee Cake Muffin) at 590 calories. The Corn Muffin and Blueberry Muffin have 460 calories each. The Honey Bran Raisin Muffin has 440 calories.

8. The correct answer is B (Beef Brisket, regular). It has 113 calories. The Turkey Breast has 142 calories; the Half Rotisserie Chicken, 341 calories; and the Pastry Top Turkey Pot Pie, 423 calories.

9. The correct answer is A (224 calories). Seafood entrees range from 30 calories for Shrimp Skewer to 510 calories for Shrimp Scampi at this restaurant.

10. The correct answer is A (Hot Chocolate) at 370 calories. The Flavored Latte has 250 calories; Cappuccino, 120 calories; and Caffe Mocha, 330 calories.

Source: Nutritional guides at restaurants, as of late 2013.

THE 17 MINUTE WORKOUT: Burning Off a Superburger

Superburgers at fast food joints can rack up almost 600 calories a serving. Here's a look at how you can burn that off.

Participate in a 90-minute aerobics dance class (five 17-minute cycles).

Jog for four 17-minute cycles.

Ride a stationary bike vigorously for four 17-minute cycles.

Shovel snow or dig ditches for three 17-minute cycles.

Walk moderately for eight 17-minute cycles (about 2½ hours).

Wouldn't it be easier not to eat the superburger?

Source: Based on research data from *Medicine and Science in Sports and Exercise,* the official journal of the American College of Sports Medicine.

Family Challenges

B eing on the 17 Day Diet can be satisfying and morale-boosting, especially as the pounds melt off. But do you ever wonder how following
the diet might affect your family at meals? You know, your loveable
hubby forcing down his baked chicken breast and green beans, missing
the dinners when fried chicken wasn't considered an outcast from the dinner table? Or your kids who are covertly trying to feed those green beans
to the family dog under the table?

A study published a few years ago in the *Journal of Nutrition Education and Behavior* looked into this issue. Researchers interviewed 21 pairs—
mostly spouses and one father-daughter duo. Their goal was to learn
whether one family member's decision to lose weight or eat healthier food
impinged on another family member's attitude or habits.

The good news is that for the most part, significant others saw themselves as positive influences on a partner's weight-loss struggles. Other
partners, however, acted badly, refusing to change their junk food habits
and, in some cases, offering little more than belittling comments. A few
doubted whether their partner could even lose weight.

Bottom line: Your loved ones—husbands, wives, your kids, even your
mother—may try to entice you to go off your diet even after you've made
it very clear you're on it. And they may not even realize they're doing this.

There are a couple of reasons why this happens. A big one is jealousy.
One person may fear that the relationship could change as a partner's
waistband gets smaller, confidence grows, and social life changes. It could
scare your spouse that you're losing weight and developing a kick-ass body.
He might fear that other men will find you attractive, and you'll leave.

People who sabotage do things like the following: Your partner might
sit down and eat a bag of cookies in front of you. Or refuse to touch your
low-fat cuisine and demand that you fix cheeseburgers. Or offer glasses of
wine, and cheese and crackers, and you fall off your weight-loss wagon
night after night. Or assign himself as the watchdog of your eating habits, telling you what to eat. This controlling attitude might backfire, mak-

ing you rebel and eat more (especially if he's not eating the same healthful way). It's nearly enough to end your commitment to diet and exercise, especially when someone's actions feel like personal attacks.

Of course, it's not just spouses or significant others who can bust up our diets. Co-workers or friends can be just as destructive and unsupportive. Even so, the biggest challenges come from right under your own roof—from your family—so that's who I really want to focus on here. Finding ways to get a partner on board is important because such support can play a major role in whether you succeed or fail.

Being the only one dieting in your family is a tough situation to be in. You make up your mind—no potato chips or chocolate ice cream in the house. No more temptations, because you're determined to change your habits and lose weight. But from talking to patients who want to lose weight, I say that's often only half the battle.

For those trying to drop pounds or eat healthier, the other half—the more trying half—can be resisting your loved ones' attempts to thwart your newfound resolve. Here are some thoughts I have on the subject.

Sabotaging Remarks and How to Respond

Don't be caught off guard by someone's remarks. Here are some suggestions for responding:

Saboteur: You're wasting away. Are you sure you aren't losing too much too fast?

You: It seems that something about me being slim is concerning you (or frightening to you or upsetting to you). But for me, my weight loss is a good and healthy thing.

Saboteur: Are you sure you can eat that?

You: My diet is varied and healthy. I eat foods in smaller portions. Or (if such comments persist): Until we can communicate about my food plan in a way that feels good to me, I don't want to discuss my diet anymore.

Saboteur: You don't like my brownies all of a sudden?

You: I like your brownies very much. But I'm not hungry right now; I'm full. (Or ask to wrap up some brownies to take home, but then toss them out.)

Saboteur: Here, one doughnut left, want it?

You: I really am working hard. I'm feeling great, and it would be nice to have your support. Is there anything I can do to help you give me that?

Saboteur: It's your birthday. One piece of cake won't hurt!

You: Yes, I know. I'm just so full . . . I'm going to take it home for later.

Saboteur: It's great you're losing weight. I hope you can keep it off this time.

You: You may feel that your comments about my weight are supportive, but it would help me if . . . (fill in the blank with something like "you didn't remind me of my past diets").

Saboteur: It's none of my business, but don't runners get a lot of knee injuries?

You: You know, I've spoken to my trainer, and my exercise habits are healthy.

Saboteur: Are you still on your diet? Have you lost any weight?

You: I appreciate your questions, but I might take them as pressure and feel frustrated if I can't report better numbers every time you ask me.

Saboteur: You know, you don't seem to be the same since you lost weight.

You: I really feel confused by that comment; I really want you to be supportive of my accomplishment.

Limit Exposure to Guy Food

Are you newly married? Some newlyweds are surprised to find out that their husbands are junk-food junkies. They love ice cream, Cheetos, dips, Oreos, and stuff you may have forgotten existed.

Exposure to guy junk food can tear down your defenses, even if you're just trying to lose 10 pounds on the 17 Day Diet. And, from my experience being a guy, I can tell you, many men do eat much more than women do, and much more of the wrong stuff. Our metabolisms are faster because we have more muscle and less fat on our bodies than you do, so many guys can burn off all the fattening garbage. It's frustrating, but let me assure you that you can lose weight while having a man under the same roof.

I believe you must set firm ground rules, like the fact that certain foods are off limits, period. Give your husband or boyfriend a special shelf (preferably one you can't reach) to stash his junk food. Or ask him to hide it. If you can't see it, you won't eat it. But don't be surprised if every now and then, you might find some Oreos in strange places, like under the sofa cushions.

Eat Less Than He Does

Men eat more than women. It's just a fact; we eat like linemen. Even the Feds have studied this: According to government surveys, the average American guy eats nearly 2,800 calories a day, while the average American gal eats around 1,800 calories a day—about a third less. If you try to keep up with him, you'll keep putting on weight. So, don't eat like he does; eat less! At restaurants, immediately put one-half of your meal to the side and bring it home in a doggie bag.

Exercise While He Watches TV

Not only do we eat like lineman, we like to watch linemen on television. If possible, place some exercise equipment in front of the television and do some time on the treadmill or stationary bike while he's watching his favorite team. This strategy will help you get thin and stay that way.

Take Charge of the Kitchen

Here is the fun part: If your husband doesn't think he likes low-fat, low-cal, healthy eating, don't worry. You can fix healthy foods by modifying his favorite recipes (don't tell him), and he'll never know the difference (except if his pants start getting mysteriously baggy and loose). Instead of using all ground beef, use ground turkey for meatloaf, for example. Make lasagna with slices of zucchini rather than with lasagna noodles. Cook vegetarian chili with tons of vegetables and beans; just don't call it vegetarian. Use cooking spray to sauté foods; it's a great way to cut down on the fat and calories. Done correctly, with the right food substitutions, low-fat meals taste as good—and sometimes better—than their fattening counterparts.

Become Fitness Pals

In all seriousness, the best strategy is to get healthy and fit together. As any expert will tell you, it's much easier to eat healthy, nonfattening food if everyone around you is too. You can make a big deal out of each others' success, congratulating yourselves the whole time. Enjoy mealtime conversations again, instead of wolfing down food. Work out together. Invite your spouse or partner to try exercising, to try this diet, or try healthy food. Phrase it lovingly: "I want to spend more time with you because I love being together. Let's do an exercise program together, like some couples' training or couples' yoga, or let's start bike riding after work. Wouldn't that be a great opportunity to be together more often?"

The decision to get fit together is a show of love and affection. Explain that healthy cooking accomplishes the same end: Healthy cooking = love. Your reformed spouse will see that coming up with nonfattening meals is a bigger present than loading you up with junk, especially when he sees all the weight you're losing and how wonderful you look. Maybe someone should think of adding a line to the wedding vows: "For richer, for poorer . . . for thinner, for fatter . . ."

By sharing the health and fitness experience with a partner, you can help each other stay motivated. Partners encourage one another to move from unhealthy to healthy behaviors. One study found that women who work out with their husbands are more likely to stick to fitness programs than married women who exercise alone. Another found that men are three times more likely to stay on a healthy diet if their wives encourage them to do so.

Sharing the fitness experience gives you something to talk about. Better communication, especially in loving relationships, is always a source of greater closeness.

DANIELLA: I Broke Through!

It was June 13, 2011, when I started the 17 day diet. I lost 100 pounds by January 13, 2012. I have lost a few more pounds and have kept it off now for 2 years. This weight loss has let me feel more comfortable with myself.

I went to the doctor for a checkup. The lab did some blood work, and found out I have hypothyroidism (sluggish thyroid). My doctor was amazed that I could have lost all that weight and kept it off with this condition.

I started out exercising just 17 minutes per day by walking 5 to 6 days a week. As I started to lose and had more energy I improved to walking 2 to 4 miles 40 to 90 minutes per day; also, I started water acrobatics.

I used many of recipes on *The Doctors* internet site. Without the special 17 Day Diet recipes, I don't think I would have stuck to it.

I kept a diary of my progress to my goal; this motivated me to stay the course.

On January 1, 2012, my husband and my son put 90 pounds on a weight bar, so I could feel the weight that I had been carrying for so long.

A friend and I have even done a couple of sets of classes at our church to help people follow this diet. Support is so important.

I have tried many diets, and they may have worked for a little while, but the weight would come back within a year. I was thinking about having surgery if this diet didn't work. But, after the first day, when I lost 5 pounds, I was hooked.

I now have the energy to do things with my family and feel I will be around now to play with my granddaughters!

The 17 Day Diet has changed my life.

Before   *After*

Find Other Supporters

If you've tried your best but can't get your husband or partner on board, seek help elsewhere, such as with a friend, a coworker, other family member, or hire a personal trainer. They can give you encouragement and inspiration. If you don't get any takers, join a group, such as a walking club or a local yoga class. These activities are fun, and you get to meet more fitness-minded people that way.

Having positive support helps you reach your dieting and fitness goals. With two or more of you working together, there's more motivation to get to your goals.

No matter how challenging your situation, stay focused and remember your reasons for wanting to get slimmer and healthier. Imagine if someone told you that you could live longer and have less pain in your life. Would you listen to what they had to say? Exercise and healthy eating is as close to the fountain of youth as we have today.

Review

- Being on a diet affects the people around you. It's important for your success to bring them on board.
- Be prepared to respond to saboteurs.
- Negotiate the presence of junk food in the house with your spouse and other family members.
- Take charge of your kitchen and learn how to cook healthy meals that everyone in your family will love.
- Invite your spouse or partner to join you in your effort to get more fit.
- Build a support group of other fitness-minded people.

MISTER M.D., CAN YOU PLEASE TELL ME

I Live Alone and Sometimes It's Hard to Stay on a Diet. What Suggestions Do You Have for Me?

Single-person households have grown from 7 percent in the sixties to 27 percent of the total today. Many single diners are deficient in calcium, iron, and other important vitamins and minerals because they skip meals, snack for dinner, or open the freezer and prepare whatever falls out. Eating alone can be a pleasurable and healthy activity, if you plan your life around it. Some suggestions:

- Stock your kitchen with a variety of staples with a long shelf-life, such as brown rice, oatmeal, and other whole grains.
- Keep on hand chopped broccoli, bagged lettuce, and yogurt, so you don't use time as an excuse not to prepare foods.

- Make single dish meals with all the components—grains, meat, and vegetables—in casseroles and soups. Prepare them ahead of time and freeze them so you don't have to cook a lot. Also, you can make the whole recipe but portion it into individual bags.

- Take advantage of supermarket salad bars. They're a boon to single people who may have avoided fresh fruits and vegetables they couldn't use fast enough. Skip the mayonnaise-based salads and high-fat dressings, but load up on fresh vegetables and fruits. At home you can add some low-fat meat or cheese, tuna, or kidney beans, and your own favorite low-fat dressing.

- Never underestimate the uses of your freezer and microwave. Bags of frozen vegetables can be a great alternative when fresh produce is not available. Rice and pasta leftovers are particularly good candidates for freezing and later use. Use your microwave for defrosting, reheating, or to speed preparation of almost any meal. Microwave dishes often can be prepared with less fat, too, by adding bouillon, wine, or broth.

- Dinner should be pleasant, and atmosphere does contribute to a more enjoyable meal. Set the table with linens, attractive dinnerware, and a centerpiece. Make a lovely meal with fresh ingredients and enjoy it with a little wine, some jazz on the stereo and a couple of candles. Sit at the table; don't just eat hanging over the sink.

- If you're single, try to get together with friends on a regular schedule. Set up a Thursday night supper club and rotate homes or try a new restaurant once a month.

- Form a cooking club with your friends. Or have a regular date to eat 17 Day Diet approved dishes with friends once a week or month.

- Partner with a friend on the 17 Day Diet. Use the recipes in this book or in the *17 Day Diet Cookbook*, and cook up whole week's worth of meals that you share.

- Use the 17 Day Diet delivery service and get single serving meals delivered directly to your home.

- Don't be afraid to eat out alone. I eat out most meals and love experimenting. I'm quite oblivious to other diners so I don't mind being stared at. I simply open my iPad and scribble, which grabs the attention of the waiters, who think I'm a restaurant critic.

13

Surviving Holidays

The holidays. It's the time of year when the zipper on your dress and the springs in your bathroom scale start getting really nervous.

That's because, for a lot of dieters, packing on pounds can be a holiday tradition. Statistics on weight gain throughout the holiday season assert that you might gain five pounds if you don't keep your hands off the pumpkin pie and figgy pudding.

I started thinking about this: A five-pound weight gain is a lot of food, if you consider that it takes 3,500 calories to gain a pound. This means you'd have to have major pig-outs on a daily basis or eat several reindeer at a buffet. You'd also have to spend the entire holiday season on the couch.

Still, it's easy to gain weight over the holidays, if you figure that the traditional holiday dinner with appetizers can weigh in at more than 3,000 calories!

How about this year we change that tradition? Commit to a holiday in which you manage not to gain any weight back before it's time to resolve to lose all that weight (and so much more) yet again.

Incidentally, by *holiday*, I mean about everything that happens from Thanksgiving to Easter, and everything in between including the sweetheart of all weight-gaining holidays, Valentine's Day. Holidays, however, do not include 99-cent Big-Mac Mondays.

Okay, with all the office parties, cocktail receptions, and dinner celebrations, can you eat, drink, be merry, stay fit, and still follow the 17 Day Diet?

Answer: Absolutely—by adhering to my easy-to-follow holiday strategies. If you do, there will be no need to make a get-fit New Year's resolution, ever again. You'll start every year in super shape.

Prediet Before the Holidays Hit

To prevent packing on holiday pounds, go on the offense with predieting. It works like this: Use the Accelerate or Activate Cycles to start trimming off a few pounds of fat before the holidays get in full swing. You can do this easily with what you've already learned from the 17 Day Diet.

Don't resort to any type of crash dieting, however, in which you fast or slash calories down to 700 or less a day. This can result in a loss of muscle, decreased strength and power, low energy, moodiness or irritability, and compromised immunity. Stick to the Accelerate or Activate Cycles for best results.

Party Plans

The hardest part, I think, is all those parties and dinners.

Around holiday time, fattening, high-calorie food is all over the place. Have you noticed? It's at your office, your mother-in-law's house, and your child's classroom. We try to fight it off, but it still assaults us. Here's what I advise for enjoying yourself, without packing on any extra pounds.

- Continue the good habit of eating breakfast during the holidays to help control cravings later on. (Sorry, eggnog isn't considered a good egg substitute.)

- Have healthy snacks on hand. Go for them before you treat yourself to the splurge stuff.

- Eat a healthy dinner before you go to a holiday party. (Also, try not to eat an unhealthy dinner when you're at the party.)

- Prepare and take your own safe, low-calorie, and low-fat foods to parties.

- Choose two or three of the healthiest appetizers you can find (a little shrimp, some veggies or fruit, etc.) and put them on a small plate or napkin, then walk away from the table. (Keep in mind this should be two or three pieces of food, not two or three napkins or plates loaded with food.)

- Be smart at the buffet table. Fill three-quarters of your plate with vegetables and fruits, the rest with protein. (Pumpkin pie and chocolate-covered strawberries don't count as the veggies or fruit.

Stacking things as high as you can is not an acceptable method for filling your plate.) Do not circle the food table like a vulture. Serve yourself, and then have a seat and enjoy yourself.

- Avoid temptation. Just say "no" to packaged holiday candies and cakes! Regift them to someone who's not dieting.

- Give yourself permission to enjoy a little of everything that is usually only available during the holidays, but do it in moderation. Indulging in small amounts of holiday treats (fruitcake being the exception) might not help you lose 20 pounds over the holidays, but it might help you from raiding the Christmas tree for edible ornaments in the middle of the night.

- Bank your calories. Accumulate a deposit of uneaten calories on the days when you know that you will be attending parties or enjoying holiday feasts. Eat a light breakfast and lunch to save calories for later. If you're careful, the large withdrawal of calories at a big dinner or event later on won't break the bank.

- Be extra good on nonparty days.

- Understand the reason for the season. Holidays are a chance to enjoy and celebrate with people you care about. Put your focus more on socializing, and less on eating.

Fill Up on Fiber

There's a supereasy, no-willpower way to stay lean during the holidays, something that most of us should be doing all year but aren't: eating more fiber. Fiber will make you feel full so you won't be grabbing candy, cookies, and fruitcake like they're going out of style. What's more, the fiber found in foods such as bran, whole-wheat products, and oats acts like bouncers in a nightclub. They grab on to the fats you eat and help kick them out of the body. That means fewer calories are left behind to be stored as fat. So, fill up on legumes, fruits, and vegetables.

Manage Alcohol Consumption

At holidays, alcohol flows freely. Keep in mind that beer, wine, and hard liquor are high in calories, however. In fact, each gram of alcohol has 7 calories, compared to 4 calories per gram for other carbs. Alcohol also stimulates your appetite. Then, there is alcohol's effect on your liver, the organ that helps drive fat-burning. With alcohol in your body, the liver has to divert to burning it off, so it has less time to burn fat. Case in point: Swiss researchers at the University of Lausanne found that if someone drinks only 3 ounces of alcohol a day, about one-third less fat will be processed.

If you want to avoid drinking alcohol and still remain social, sip on seltzers, club soda, or sparkling mineral water on the rocks with a citrus twist. Or opt for nonalcoholic beer or wine. But don't overdo it, because most of these products are high in sugar.

SCIENCE SAYS: Log What You Eat, Lop Off Pounds

During the holidays, keep track of what you eat and how many calories you consume daily by writing the information down in a food journal. Termed as *self-monitoring*, this practice has been shown in research to promote weight loss, even during the holidays.

In one study, 38 dieters (32 women and 6 men) recorded their food and calorie intake during Thanksgiving, Christmas or Hanukkah, and New Year's Eve. The researchers categorized the dieters into groups according to how consistently they kept track of their food and calorie consumption. Weight loss was recorded as well. The best and most consistent self-monitors lost an average of 10 pounds more than the persons who had a low level of compliance with the monitoring program.

Fit in Exercise

The holidays are not a time to take a vacation from your workouts. Stick to your regular exercise routine. It's one of the best ways to fight fat gain during the holidays. It helps to burn off the extra calories that you've eaten at those parties and holiday get-togethers. Some ideas: Extend the duration of your usual cardio activity, or try something new, like a Zumba class.

Or just be active in other ways: go roller skating, ice skating, play racquet ball, or go skiing.

If you're not that adventurous, try to slightly increase the duration and/or frequency of your usual cardio. By *duration*, I am referring to how long you work out. You'll burn additional calories by pushing your body just a little longer.

Another option is increasing exercise frequency: working out more times per week to incinerate more calories and fat. Add some extra weekly sessions to your normal exercise routine.

Don't plop down on the sofa this holiday season—move your body!

Get a Grip on Holiday Stress

I've always thought the concept of *stress* attached to the word *holiday* was the ultimate contradiction. Shouldn't a holiday be simply filled with joy and celebration?

Yes! Even so there is holiday stress, much of it self-imposed. What is supposed to be a time of joy and good cheer begins to resemble frantic preparations for a military invasion.

Along with the season's celebrations come situations that can stress you out and make you feel draggy. And, so, you turn to food for relief. It's no wonder you often gain weight during holidays. To help you avoid all this, namely weight gain, fatigue, and stress, I'll give you my thoughts on how to organize your life to make time for what really matters. Don't let your holidays be downers. With some organization and planning, you can sail through the season with your health and emotional well-being intact, and maybe even a few pounds lighter.

- Manage your time and priorities. To prevent being hijacked by the demands of the season, do some planning. Decide which events and activities are most important and mark your calendar accordingly, along with planning for some personal time. Holidays are about family and friends, so spend more time with them. Buying presents and sending holiday cards can be overwhelming tasks. Don't try to do this all at once. Break it down into smaller amounts of time. Write out a few cards each evening, for example. I'm a busy guy myself, so I do my holiday shopping online. That way, gifts can be gift-wrapped and sent directly to my family and friends. Buying gifts online helps me avoid the annual mall death march through toy stores, factory outlets, and discount palaces.

- Guard your sleep. Stress management and overall health demand adequate sleep and should top your priority list. The best way to ensure proper rest is to set regular bedtimes. Avoid or cut down on caffeine, alcohol, and tobacco; all disrupt sleeping patterns, making it difficult to drift off or stay there. Eating too much food close to bedtime adversely affects slumber as well.

- Set reasonable goals over the holidays. If you want to shed fat, the holidays may not be the best time to do it. There are just too many tempting goodies around. In fact, a better, more reasonable goal would be to maintain your weight and not gain any.

- Cancel the guilt trips. If, after all of your planning and commitment, you do overindulge, try not to feel guilty. Guilt only weakens your resolve to maintain healthy habits. Besides, guilt can spoil the fun of your holiday celebrations, and this is a time of year to be merry. Even if you do veer off your program, don't let that be your downfall. See the bigger picture, without obsessing over every little deviation from your plan. Simply do the next healthy thing for yourself: exercise, have a nutritious meal, or do some relaxation exercises.

- Be of good cheer. Send a contribution to someone in need, volunteer at a shelter, or contribute to a charity like Toys for Tots. Take a few moments of each day to simply say thank you for what you have. Release anger, bitterness, and resentment. Be like a kid again in how you view the holidays; it will help you live with more wonder and enthusiasm. And, finally, hold each day sacred. The present is the greatest gift of all.

If you take just a few pieces of my advice, I doubt if you'll have even one vision of a sugar plum or be tempted to sneak a nibble of the carolers' figgy pudding.

Review

- Prediet prior to the holidays. That way, you'll come into the season weighing less. Should you gain weight over the holidays, it won't be such a big deal.

- Eat strategically at parties and holiday gatherings so you don't go overboard.

- Fill up on fiber-rich foods to keep from overeating.

- Keep track of what you eat during the holidays by writing it down.

- Don't neglect exercise.

- Use stress-reducing techniques during the holidays.

- Remember the real reason behind the season.

LEAN 17: The 17 Most Fattening Holiday Foods and How to Downsize Them

Here are 17 holiday favorites from around the world. Note how they stack up calorie wise, and what you can do to soften the blow.

Food	Calories per Serving	The Leaner Eat
1. 8-ounce cheese ball	729	Opt for reduced-calorie cheese as an appetizer.
2. Eggnog (9 ounces)	343	Make your own low-fat version with egg substitute, evaporated skim milk, rum extract, and some Truvia for sweetness.
3. Dinner rolls	84 to 201	Serve whole-wheat rolls or no bread at all.
4. Cranberry sauce (½ cup)	223	Serve reduced-sugar cranberry sauce and save around 150 calories.
5. Candied yams (1 cup)	420	Mash sweet potatoes with a little orange juice; skip the sugar and marshmallows.

Food	Calories per Serving	The Leaner Eat
6. Mashed potatoes and gravy, large helping	240	Mash the potatoes with 2 parts potatoes and 1 part mashed parsnips, carrots, or cauliflower to reduce the calories by nearly 75 percent. Use a little evaporated skim milk and forgo the butter. Skip or go easy on the gravy.
7. Potato pancakes (latkes), 2 pancakes	400	Use vegetable cooking spray rather than oil, and substitute egg whites for the eggs.
8. Creamed corn (1 cup)	184	Enjoy regular cooked corn kernels instead.
9. Traditional stuffing, large serving	640	Substitute brown rice for bread, and bake it separately in a covered casserole. When cooked inside the turkey, the stuffing absorbs gobs of unhealthy fat from the turkey.
10. Roast goose	519	Stick with roast turkey.
11. Prime rib	569 to 854, depending on the size of the slab	Control your portion size!
12. Roast pork with pineapple	466	Roast a pork loin (it is a lean cut of pork) in the oven by removing the skin, draining the fat, and adding broth, fruit, or bitter orange or orange juice instead of oil to keep it moist. Serve with pineapple canned in its own juice in order to avoid added sugar.
13. Tamales, 3	459	Rather than using lard or shortening, make the tamales with a healthier vegetable oil, such as olive or canola. You can also save fat and calories by making them vegetarian with a Mexican cheese or Monterey

		Jack and adding a green chili (jalapeño or Anaheim, for example) for an extra kick.
14. Lasagna, beef, 1 piece	377	Prepare vegetable lasagna and enjoy 1 piece instead of 2. Or make lasagna the American way with lean ground beef, part-skim mozzarella, fat-free Parmesan cheese, and low-fat ricotta cheese.
15. Pecan pie, 1 slice (1/8 of a 9" pie)	503	Pumpkin pie is a better bet. Some weigh in at only 150 calories per slice.
16. Apple pie, 1 slice (1/8 of a 9" pie)	411	Go for pumpkin pie instead.
17. Christmas cookies	200	It's okay if you eat one, but who can stop at one?

MISTER M.D., CAN YOU PLEASE TELL ME

I Love The Holidays, but I Eat Too Many Sweets and Can't Stop. Why?

Sweet foods really do make you hungry. The more sweets you eat, the more you crave them. Why? When you eat sugary stuff, your blood sugar soars. Insulin then enters the picture to bring it down, by ushering sugar into cells for energy, and fast. Then there's a corresponding drop in blood sugar, a plummet that increases your appetite, and you might start craving sweets even more.

You've just got to cut back or avoid them altogether, and the cravings will ease up and may even disappear. Put off going grocery shopping during the holidays. The fattening stuff in your fridge will disappear first. After a few days, the cookies, ice cream, and pecan pie are history. All that's left are the raw vegetables. This can force you to eat a healthy diet. If you procrastinate long enough before going grocery shopping, you might have to end up eating a raw beet. My point is: out of sight, out of mind. If holiday treats are calling your name, keep them out of earshot—which means out of your house.

GET SKINNY SHORTCUT

No sweets from your sweetie. Candy may be dandy for romance, but it can mean love handles in a hurry. Just about everyone likes candy during Valentine's Day, but did you know that those small pieces of chocolate contain about 70 to 150 calories each? Thinking about snacking on the box? Not so fast. An average box of candy can contain 10,000 calories or more. And as far as timing goes, by Valentine's Day, most people are still trying to get rid of the excess pounds they put on during Christmas and New Year's. And before that came all the Halloween candy. Ask your sweetie to romance you with flowers, perfume, or a special spa day.

14

The 17 Day Diet on the Road

I once had a patient—I'll call her Tina—who flew occasionally. She was about 5'9"and weighed 155, not too bad for her height.

Then she was hired for a job that required a lot of air travel. Tina liked to travel. However, the travel interfered with her exercise and diet. Weight kept creeping on. At the end of the year, she had gained 5 pounds. Same chapter, same verse the next year. Although she loved her job and wasn't going to quit it, she did not like the 25-plus pounds she had gained. So, she used the 17 Day Diet to reverse the trend. She was successful, even though she continues flying 100,000 miles a year. She keeps her weight off by using the strategies I'll give you here. I've got some advice that I'm convinced will work for you as you take off weight while occupying the friendly skies, and elsewhere on your travels.

At the Airport

Let's be honest: Most airport eateries aren't noted for the variety or quality of their offerings. Airports are filled with high-fat, high-sugar snacks. If I must chew on something, I stroll right past the kiosks selling junk food and look for places where I can buy fruit, low-fat yogurt, or a salad.

Carefully examine the menu in airport restaurants. You can usually find a low-fat or low-calorie selection. If you have to grab airport food, look for a way to bulk up your fiber intake with things like fresh fruit (especially berries), salads, whole grains, and vegetable soups.

What if you can't find anything that qualifies as healthful? Sometimes I simply go hungry a while longer. If I must order a less-than-healthful item, I eat only a small portion of it. (Be warned: This tactic requires extraordinary willpower.)

Be active. Avoid the moving walkway. Unless you're absolutely going to miss a connecting flight, walk briskly to your next gate using your own two feet without the mechanical help.

Walk the concourse. If you have time between connecting flights, start walking around at a comfortably fast pace. Sure, I know you might be tired after a long flight and don't want to trudge through the airport, pulling your carry-on through throngs of other passengers. But, trust me, a little walk will rejuvenate you and prevent travel pounds from piling on. Try to get in at least 10 to 20 minutes of brisk walking.

On the Plane

Airline food is almost universally considered a bad dining experience. We've all seen those UFOs (unidentified fried objects) and had that ubiquitous chicken breast which has circumnavigated the globe many times by now. If you're on a flight that offers a meal service (or you're fortunate enough to have upgraded to a class that provides an actual meal), make the same choices you would in a restaurant. Choose the low-calorie, low-fat, healthful selections, and eat sparingly of those carb-rich items like rolls and desserts. Also, use only half the salad dressing you're given, and don't put butter on the roll. Ask if you can have some fresh fruit as a substitute for dessert. Little things add up fast.

Try to eat like you would at home. So, if you don't tend to polish off a three-course meal with a giant hot fudge sundae at home, don't eat one on the plane. I guarantee it's not going to be the best hot fudge sundae you've ever had, so why blow it on something mediocre?

Don't drink too many calories. When the beverage cart rolls your way, ask for water, tomato juice, or a calorie-free diet drink. Just say no to alcohol and beverages with caffeine because they contribute to dehydration. The snacks-for-purchase on flights aren't the greatest, so pass those up, too. I suggest bringing your own healthy stuff to snack on: fresh fruits, cut-up veggies, or one of my Power Cookies.

On long flights, move around from time to time. I don't mean roam the aisle and get in the flight attendants' way. Just stand up every half-hour or so and stretch your legs, arms, and other muscles.

This doesn't just burn a few calories; it may help prevent deep-vein thrombosis (DVT), a serious medical complication of long flights. If your legs are immobile for long periods, blood can gather in the lower limbs and form a clot in the veins found in the muscles. If the clot then travels to the heart, lungs, or brain, it can be fatal. You're more at risk of a deep-vein thrombosis if you're elderly, obese, have conditions such as cancer, or another acute medical illness, and if you have undergone surgery, or are pregnant, on birth control pills, or hormone replacement therapy.

There are other preventive measures you can take if you're at risk. A 20 to 30 minute brisk walk around the terminal building will keep your circulation going over several hours. Stay hydrated, too. Alcohol dehydrates you and makes you less mobile, increasing the risk of blood clots. Lots of airlines now offer exercise routines that you can do in your seat.

Traveling by Car

Don't forget your cooler, and pack your own meals, including low-fat snacks. Choose 98 percent fat-free lunch meats, fresh fruits and vegetables, and water. Enjoy the trip by stopping at rest areas instead of fast-food chains. When eating at fast-food chains, choose from the menu wisely. Skip the French fries and mayonnaise. Go for the salads.

Food at the Hotel

Arriving late at night at your hotel? You might be tempted to call room service, but fight that urge! Eating too late at night is detrimental to weight control, because you can't burn it off while you're sleeping. And the mini-bar? Don't even think about it!

Staying nutritionally healthy on the road can be challenging, because you'll be eating out a lot. What I like to do is go online and research restaurants in a city or town to identify which ones offer healthy choices. Then make a list of where to find the healthiest breakfasts, lunches, and dinners, and remember to stay away from the all-you-can-eat joints.

Start Your Day Healthy

I've found that if I start my travel day out with good choices, like a veggie egg white omelet or a bowl of oatmeal with fruit, then I make healthy choices the rest of the day. Of course, above all, stay hydrated. Keep bottles of water on hand to prevent thirst and to curb hunger (since hunger often masks as thirst).

LEAN 17: 17 Packable, Travel-Worthy Snacks

1. 4 oz. applesauce cups (unsweetened)

2. Fat-free pudding snack cups

3. 4 oz. fruit cups, packed in fruit juice

4. Apple or pear

5. My Lean Granola

6. My Power Cookie

7. Cut up raw veggies: carrots, celery, sugar-snap peas, pepper, or cucumber strips

8. Baby carrots

9. Single-serve box of high-fiber cereal

10. String cheese

11. One boiled egg

12. Small bag of fat-free popcorn

13. Small bag of grapes

14. Healthy sandwich with veggies

15. Beef or turkey jerky

16. Orange

17. Edamame

Exercising on the Road

I like to make reservations at a hotel with an exercise room, preferably one that's open around the clock. This has become a must have for me. The only way I'll break that rule is if I have no other choice (for example, if I have to stay at a specific hotel in connection with a medical convention or meeting I'm attending).

If the hotel doesn't have a fitness room, there may be a nearby gym where you can get a one-day pass for a small fee. Once you get there, try their classes. It can be fun to experience a new gym or a new class in another city.

I like to exercise in the morning. That way, I get it over with. At the end of a travel day there are too many situations that may get in the way. Besides, if I work out in the morning, I feel better the rest of the day.

Be creative. Most hotel rooms have enough floor space to allow you to turn your room into a minigym. Pack workout DVDs or jump ropes. Stack phone books for a step workout performed to a favorite exercise video.

Pack some resistance bands. You can work your whole body with this versatile piece of equipment, and in a relatively small space.

But don't forget bodyweight exercises like push-ups, sit-ups, or squats or lunges with some luggage in hand. Also, tune into exercise shows on television and join right in.

Mix business and pleasure. Find a local club where you can dance. It's an easy way to burn calories and check out the nightlife.

Don't forget to pack your swimsuit. If your hotel has a pool, dive in and do laps. Swimming works every muscle in the body and is a great way to relieve stress.

Another strategy I like is to ask for a room on the second floor or higher, so you can use the stairs in the hotel for a great workout. Mark off 17 minutes on your watch. Walk down the hall of the hotel to the stairs. Walk up a floor, then down the hallway of that floor. Go up another floor and walk that hallway. Continue in this manner for 8½ minutes, then repeat the course down and back to your room. Just make sure you get back to the right floor, and the right room. I've made that mistake before. It's not a pretty picture, trying to get in a room that's not yours.

Also, I bypass the elevator even if I'm carrying luggage and my room is located on the 12th floor. It's amazing how much heart-pumping cardio action you can get from climbing the stairs instead of taking the elevator. In some hotels, taking the stairs will get you to your room faster than the elevator will.

If stairs aren't your thing, consider the outdoors. How about seeing the sights by walking, hiking, or renting a bike? Ask the local bike shop about the best and safest routes. Walking is a great way to explore new places and stay fit while doing it. It's my favorite travel workout. Ask the hotel concierge for suggestions of walkable routes. Walking to your destination can also save on taxi fares.

Whew. I just think I burned 1,000 calories writing about all that.

So many people tell me they can't stay fit while traveling, but I don't buy it—that just means they don't want it badly enough. Good planning helps you fit fitness into your travel plans.

Review

- Make healthy choices at airports or on planes.
- Use the airport as a gym if you have time. Walk the concourse for exercise.
- Choose wisely at hotels, and when dining out.
- Start your day healthy with a nutritious breakfast and exercise.
- Book a hotel with a fitness center, or turn your hotel room into a gym.
- Handle vacations by keeping up your exercise program, planning for special dietary needs, focusing on nonfood aspects of the vacation, and making healthy choices.

HOW TO HANDLE VACATIONS

"Would you like soup and salad to go with your meal?"

"What would you like for dessert?"

"Where should we eat today?"

"Let's hit the midnight buffet."

Recently, I was bombarded with these questions while on vacation. I was being offered 12-course meals, all-you-can-eat breakfast and lunch buffets, and a grill that was open 24 hours a day.

But after days and days of enjoying delicious foods, I realized that vacations do not mean diet disaster. Vacations mean enjoying yourself while maintaining your weight. Yes, they present additional challenges when you are trying to lose weight and maintain an exercise program. An example I hear over and over again from people is: "I love going on cruises, but every time I do, I end up triggering myself to fall off my program for the rest of the year."

In cases like this, what should you do? I'd never suggest that you stop going on cruises, all-inclusive vacations, or other destinations where food is so prevalent. I might propose that you look for ways to be more active on one of these vacations, plan to make healthier food choices, or replace one of your yearly vacations with another type of vacation that is more active.

Vacations are not incompatible with watching your diet. They can always fit right into your lifestyle, and you don't have to overeat every time you go out of town or enjoy a holiday. There are always alternatives. Here are some practical suggestions to help you through vacations without undoing all the hard work you have put into losing weight:

- Decide on your goal over the vacation. Do you want to maintain your current weight or continue to keep losing weight? For weight loss, you'll have to monitor your calorie intake; if maintaining your weight is your goal, then you can adjust your calories upward slightly.

- If you have special dietary needs, plan accordingly. Some cruise lines, for example, offer heart-healthy meals low in fat and sodium and allow special orders.

- Focus on the other enjoyable aspects of the vacation, rather than the food—the locale, the sightseeing, and the activities.

- Make healthy food choices as much as possible, with an emphasis on fruits, vegetables, whole grains, and lean proteins. To keep your hunger in check, lean toward high-fiber foods and foods with a high water content, such as raw or steamed whole vegetables and fruits. A sensible approach can help you avoid overeating.

- Make special requests for food that may not be on the menu. Many resorts offer these types of dietary accommodations.

- Keep an eye on your serving sizes and always practice portion control.

- Join the walking, aerobics, and dancing programs when you're on a cruise or at a resort, and use the exercise equipment in the gym. Take the most active shore excursions, or visit ports of call on your own and use guidebooks to create your own walking tour.

- Sightseeing activities get the muscles moving, but choose a tour that allows you opportunities to exercise. For example, time on your own in a city means you can jog or take a vigorous walk to attractions and shops. Ask whether the lodgings on a tour have lap pools or exercise rooms. If you happen to splurge, get back on course right away, whether this means taking a short walk or eating one healthy meal. Congratulate yourself for getting back on your program and acting in a healthy manner. After doing this a few times, you'll develop a positive mind-set and begin to believe you can accomplish whatever it is you want.

Shift Work on the 17 Day Diet

I 'm sure you've heard the song, "Nine to Five." It has catchy lyrics, but they don't describe the real-life experience of about 15 million Americans. That's how many shift workers—on duty evenings, nights, or in some rotating or otherwise irregular schedule—the U.S. Bureau of Labor Statistics estimates are in the workforce. And you may be one of them. Occupations affected include: the military, food services, transportation, manufacturing industry, police, firefighters, security personnel, and health-care providers.

Unlike nocturnal animals, such as owls and mice, most humans have some trouble adjusting to this strange lifestyle of working at night and sleeping during the day. This is because shift work, including night work, disrupts the body's *circadian rhythm*—the internal clock that regulates when to eat and sleep; raises and lowers body temperature; and runs other regular biological processes, all hardwired and regulated to the rising and setting of the sun.

Tinkering with that clock can have some serious consequences on your weight. Shift workers have a higher prevalence of being overweight—a fact substantiated by research. There are four main reasons.

First, regular eating and exercise habits are tough to maintain on shift work. You can get bored easily, so you tend to nibble on junk food. According to a study by the New York Obesity Research Center, published in *Nutrition* in 2000, late-shift workers gained an average of 9.5 pounds during their late-shift tenure, while their day-shift counterparts gained only 2 pounds.

Second, there's a hormonal issue. When you sleep and eat at irregular times, your metabolism gets thrown out of whack. At night, during sleep, your body's insulin-making processes naturally go into hibernation. You're not eating, so the body doesn't require much insulin to process glucose from food. But if you eat on your night shift, there's not much insulin action so your body drives nutrients toward fat accumulation this late in the day.

Third, digestive problems are at fault. Shift workers have nearly double the digestive problems as their counterparts on the day shift. During nighttime, your digestive system thinks it's time to snooze and doesn't behave normally. Plus, your metabolism slows down in the evening. Many shift workers report nasty gastrointestinal symptoms such as diarrhea, constipation, ulcers, and nausea.

Finally, there are sleep problems. Shift workers are probably the most sleep-deprived folks in the country. Think about it: It's got to be tough to sleep 8 hours during the day, when your body clock thinks you should be wide awake. Also, sleep deprivation drives down *leptin*, a hormone produced in fat cells that tells your brain when you're full. At the same time, your substandard snoozing causes a rise in *ghrelin*, a hormone that makes you feel like you haven't eaten since two Mondays ago. Numerous studies showed that those who sleep less than eight hours a night have lower levels of leptin, higher levels of ghrelin, and more body fat than the long-slumbering subjects. Chronic sleep deprivation can thus drastically increase your risk of gaining weight.

The weird hours you have as a shift worker have a bunch of nutritional land mines—so here are some ways to avoid diet traps, stay true to the 17 Day Diet, and keep your body in super shape.

Avoid Junk Food

Here's something I learned on my shift work as an intern and resident: The better you eat on your shift, the more energy you'll have and the more alert you'll be. First rule here: If it comes out of a vending machine, it's off limits. There's mostly junk food behind that glass, and it will do nothing for your weight or energy levels.

The same goes for drinks: No sodas for you! Go easy on the caffeine, too, because you'll find it harder to get shut-eye when you get home. The very best beverage you can drink on your shift is water. It will keep you hydrated and energized.

On night shift, the best meals to eat are light ones. A too-full tummy can make you drag. Populate those meals with lots of raw fruits and veggies, as recommended on the 17 Day Diet. These will give you energy but won't make you sleepy.

Sometimes shifts are eight hours or longer with overtime, so you need foods that will help sustain your energy levels. Some examples: sandwiches made with lean meat and whole-grain or gluten-free bread. The combo of protein and whole-grains will make you feel full and less likely to snack. As for gluten-free bread, the older we get, the tougher it is for our bodies to digest gluten. It can block the bowel and make things more sluggish. A healthy bowel that moves things along gives you much more energy.

Follow My Sample Shift Menus

Let's put these suggestions in concrete form. All cycles of the 17 Day Diet are adaptable to shift work. It just takes a little bit of planning. If possible, eat your 17 Day Diet meals at approximately the same time each day, either at noon or in the early evening, whether you are on the night shift or not. Follow these guidelines, and you'll get in better sync, lose weight, and be more alert.

Sample Shift Menu: Afternoon Shift (Starting between 2:00 and 4:00 p.m.; finishing between 10:00 p.m. and midnight)

Generally, if you work an afternoon shift, it's best to have your main meal in the middle of the day rather than in the middle of your shift. You'll burn off your food better and stay more alert on your shift.

Here are some meal-planning suggestions for each cycle.

Time of Day/Meal	Accelerate Cycle	Activate Cycle	Achieve Cycle	Arrive Cycle
8:00 to 10:00 a.m./ Breakfast	2 scrambled eggs, fresh fruit, 6 oz. yogurt	½ cup oatmeal or grits, cooked; 4 egg whites, scrambled; fresh fruit	1 cup cereal, high-fiber (i.e., Bran Buds or Fiber One); 1 cup (8 oz.) skim, 1%, or soy milk or other dairy substitute; fresh fruit	Stick to whole grains and protein.

Time of Day/Meal	Accelerate Cycle	Activate Cycle	Achieve Cycle	Arrive Cycle
1:00 to 2:00 p.m. Dinner (before shift)	Grilled chicken breast with liberal amounts of any vegetables, steamed or raw; fresh fruit	Pork sirloin chops, broiled or grilled; steamed veggies; ½ cup cooked corn; 6 oz. yogurt or other probiotic serving; fresh fruit	Grilled chicken; steamed vegetables such as asparagus, wax beans, broccoli, or cauliflower; fresh fruit	Focus on protein-rich foods; they keep you alert.
7:00 to 8:00 p.m. Lunch at work	Tuna tossed with 1 tablespoon olive oil and a tablespoon of vinegar, served over a generous bed of lettuce; 6 oz. yogurt or other probiotic serving to help with digestion	Shrimp salad: cooked shrimp, 3 tablespoons chopped onion, generous bed of lettuce leaves, 1 tomato (large) and 1 tablespoon olive oil; 6 oz. yogurt or other probiotic serving to help with digestion	Pita sandwich: 1 whole-wheat pita filled with chopped lettuce and tomato; 2 tablespoons crumbled fat-free feta cheese; 1 tablespoon Italian salad dressing; 10 baby carrots; 6 oz. yogurt or other probiotic serving to help with digestion	Continue focusing on protein-rich foods. Munch on fresh fruit and vegetables. Don't overload yourself on carbs. Be sure to include probiotic foods to help with digestion.

Time of Day/Meal	Accelerate Cycle	Activate Cycle	Achieve Cycle	Arrive Cycle
After work/ before bedtime	Have some fresh fruit.	Have a carb or two. Bananas are a good choice because they help with sleep.	Have a carb or two. Bananas are a good choice because they help with sleep.	Have a carb or two. Bananas are a good choice because they help with sleep.

Sample Shift Menu: Night Shift (Midnight to 8:00 a.m.)

Generally, night-shift workers should snack lightly during their shift, eat a moderate breakfast, and have dinner before their shift starts.

Here's a look at how to plan your diet.

Time of Day/Meal	Accelerate Cycle	Activate Cycle	Achieve Cycle	Arrive Cycle
When you wake up	2 scrambled eggs, fresh fruit, 6 oz. yogurt	½ cup oatmeal or grits, cooked; 4 egg whites, scrambled; fresh fruit	1 cup cereal, high-fiber (i.e. Bran Buds or Fiber One); 1 cup (8 oz.) skim, 1%, or soy milk or other dairy substitute; fresh fruit	Egg-white omelet with tomatoes; one slice of whole-wheat toast with jam; ½ cup of fresh strawberries; tea, coffee, or water

Time of Day/Meal	Accelerate Cycle	Activate Cycle	Achieve Cycle	Arrive Cycle
6:00 to 8:00 p.m./ Dinner (before shift)	Grilled chicken breast with liberal amounts of any vegetables, steamed or raw; fresh fruit	Pork sirloin chops, broiled or grilled; steamed veggies; ½ cup cooked corn	Grilled chicken; steamed vegetables such as asparagus, wax beans, broccoli, or cauliflower; fresh fruit	Dinner: green salad with salad veggies, oil and vinegar dressing; broiled chicken breast with lemon and rosemary; ½ cup of brown rice; steamed broccoli; fresh fruit cup; water
3:00 to 4:00 a.m. Lunch at work	Tuna tossed with 1 tablespoon olive oil and a tablespoon of vinegar, served over a generous bed of lettuce; 6 oz. yogurt or other probiotic serving to help with digestion	Shrimp salad: cooked shrimp, 3 tablespoons chopped onion, generous bed of lettuce leaves, 1 tomato (large), and 1 tablespoon olive oil; 6 oz. yogurt or other probiotic serving to help with digestion	Pita sandwich: 1 whole-wheat pita filled with chopped lettuce and tomato; 2 tablespoons crumbled fat-free feta cheese; 1 tablespoon Italian salad dressing; 10 baby carrots; 6 oz. yogurt or other probiotic serving to help with digestion	Green salad with avocado and 4 oz. of steamed salmon, oil and vinegar dressing. Iced tea or water; 6 oz. yogurt or other probiotic serving to help with digestion.

Time of Day/Meal	Accelerate Cycle	Activate Cycle	Achieve Cycle	Arrive Cycle
After shift, before sleep	Have some fresh fruit.	Have a carb or two. Bananas are a good choice because they help with sleep.	Have a carb or two. Bananas are a good choice because they help with sleep.	Have a carb or two. Bananas are a good choice because they help with sleep.

LEAN 17: 17 Foods that Keep You Alert

Most of the foods on the 17 Day Diet can help you stay more alert and are perfect for shift work. Choose more of the following foods if you're a shift worker.

Food	Alertness Factor
1. Beef, extra lean	High in iron, a mineral that improves memory, alertness, and attention span.
2. Beets	Contain *phenylalanine*, an amino acid that helps relay signals from one brain cell to another.
3. Blueberries	Excellent source of antioxidants and *anthocyanins*, compounds thought to help protect brain cells from toxins, improves use of glucose in the brain, and promotes communication between brain cells.
4. Broccoli	Packed with antioxidants and phytonutrients that help protect brain tissue from toxins.
5. Carrots	High in beta carotene and other natural substances that help protect brain tissue from toxins.
6. Chicken	High in tyrosine, an amino acid required for the production of the alertness chemicals dopamine, epinephrine, and norepinephrine. When your brain is producing these, you think and react more quickly, and feel more motivated, attentive, and mentally energetic.
7. Citrus fruits	Contain vitamin C and other antioxidants that help maintain sharp memory and help brain cells resist damage.

8. Edamame	Contains *phenylalanine*, an amino acid that helps relay signals from one brain cell to another.
9. Eggs	High in the B vitamin *choline*, which helps with memory.
10. Egg whites	High in protein, which can improve alertness by increasing levels of *norepinephrine*, which helps keep your brain at its sharpest.
11. Hot chilies	Contain the fiery-tasting chemical capsaicin. Capsaicin stimulates circulation, aids digestion, opens your nasal passages, and, even better, sends a feeling of euphoria straight to your brain.
12. Legumes	Provide glucose to fuel the brain, and the fiber they contain slows the absorption of glucose, helping to maintain stable levels of energy and support alertness and concentration over time.
13. Pork	Loaded with vitamin B1, which protects *myelin*, a fatty substance that helps facilitate communication among cells.
14. Romaine lettuce	High in *folate*, a B vitamin important for memory and nerve cell health.
15. Spinach	Packed with iron, which is involved memory, concentration, and mental functioning.
16. Tuna	Full of omega-3 fatty acids, which help build and maintain myelin.
17. Yogurt	A probiotic food that has been found in many studies to boost mental alertness. Yogurt and other probiotic foods are great foods for night shift work, since they help your digestion.

The Exercise Connection

Let's look on the bright side of the night shift: You get to go to the gym while almost everybody else is at work. Try picking a good time early in your day. Even if you do only half your usual workout, you'll be moving your body, and you'll feel better. Seventeen minutes of exercise at least three times each week (though not just before bedtime) will help reduce stress, make you more energetic, and enhance your sense of well-being.

Be consistent with your training and add in some fun cross-training activities. You might have more time for outdoor bicycle rides, for example, with your night-shift schedule. As you catch up on your sleep, train longer and/or harder until you're back to your former training level.

Sleep Sense

If you work when everyone else is snoozing, you win: You don't have to mess with commuter traffic, you get to be around when your kids get home, and often night shift folks get a bigger paycheck. It's not all bad, and I know a lot of people who prefer the night shift!

However, you may not get the seven to eight hours of shut-eye most of us need, and that's dangerous for your health, your weight, and for other drivers if you're feeling pooped behind the wheel.

Trying to sleep during the day can present a challenge, especially if family members are rattling around in the kitchen and kids are coming and going. I can't give you a surefire recipe for sound sleep during the day, but I have several techniques that should help. Even if each technique helps you sleep only a little better, all together they may let you get the rest you deserve and need.

One key strategy is to maintain a somewhat constant schedule. Don't sleep from noon to 8:00 p.m. on Friday, then try sleeping nights on Saturday and Sunday, then switch back to day sleeping on Monday. Even if you alter your schedule somewhat, don't change too much. A study in the *New Zealand Journal of Psychology* advises a strategy called *anchor sleep*, in which you include a three- to four-hour block of sleep time on non-shift-work days that coincides with your anticipated sleep time on shift-work days.

Get to bed as soon as possible after the night shift. If you don't sleep after the night shift, your body clock will get you ready for daytime. Darken your bedroom. You want the place in which you're sleeping to be as dark as possible. Consider blackout curtains or shades, a sleep mask, or anything else that reduces light. This is vital, since *melatonin*, the hormone of sleep that increases drowsiness, is suppressed by daylight, even through closed eyelids. Light leaks through, then sets your brain's internal clock. You've got to fool your brain into believing that day is night, and vice versa. No light? Your brain says it must be night.

Sleep in a quiet room in your house, away from outside noise and household commotion. Tell family and friends about your shift schedule, and ask them to get in touch with you only during your waking hours.

Moderate your use of caffeine. Many of us toss back coffee to keep up energy at work. Not a good idea. It's tempting for night workers to drink a lot of coffee at the end of their shifts because it's when they're most sluggish, but that's only likely to continue to interfere with sleep quality.

Eat a banana or sip some warm milk prior to bedtime. Both these foods are high in *l-tryptophan*, an amino acid thought to be a natural sleeping pill. L-tryptophan releases *serotonin*, a sleep-inducing brain chemical.

Stay away from alcohol prior to sleep. It is a diuretic that will make you go to the bathroom when you need to be snoozing in the bedroom. Also, alcohol interferes with the quality of your sleep.

Try an herbal tea prior to bedtime. Teas containing valerian root can be a safe, effective way to sleep when you really need to. As with any sleep aid, it should be used sparingly, however. Some people feel groggy upon awakening if they've taken valerian. (The best sleep aid is regular exercise.)

If you're a shift worker, you have to take extra care of yourself. It's worth your quality of life and livelihood to do so.

Review

- Shift workers suffer from obesity and other illnesses more often than people who work regular shifts.

- If you're a shift worker, avoid junk food. Have your main meal in the middle of the day if you work an afternoon shift, and have dinner just before your shift starts if you work the midnight shift.

- Populate your night with natural foods that keep you alert.

- Maintain a consistent exercise schedule.

- Practice good sleep health: Keep your bedroom as dark as possible, sleep in a quiet part of your house, limit your use of caffeine and alcohol, and have a snack such as a banana and some warm milk prior to going to bed.

- Talk to your family doctor if you think you might be suffering from shift work disorder.

CHECK-UP: Do You Have Shift Work Disorder?

The term *shift work disorder*, or SWD, may be unfamiliar to you, but it's getting a lot of attention. If you work an afternoon or night shift, and are often tired on the job or have trouble sleeping, it's a condition you should learn more about.

SWD is now a recognized medical condition, and it can be diagnosed and treated by a physician. It occurs when your body's internal clock is not synchronized with your work schedule. Put another way: Your body thinks it should be sleeping when you are actually awake, on the job and working. Being out of sync like this can make you feel very sleepy during your waking hours, and you might have trouble falling asleep when you need to. If you're a shift worker, take the following quiz to see if you might have shift work disorder. Circle either "yes" or "no."

1. Do you feel tired no matter how much sleep you try to get?   Yes   No

2. Are you often less alert than you could be?   Yes   No

3. Do you have difficulty falling asleep or staying asleep?   Yes   No

4. Are you unaware of your total sleeping hours per day?   Yes   No

5. Have you been making more errors at work than usual
   due to lack of focus and general sense of fatigue?   Yes   No

6. Do you frequently suffer from heartburn or indigestion?   Yes   No

7. Do you experience occasional morning headaches?   Yes   No

8. Has your work, home, or social life been negatively
   affected by sleeping problems?   Yes   No

9. Have you been experiencing unexplained weight gain?   Yes   No

10. Have you been experiencing irregular menstrual cycles?   Yes   No

11. Do you feel very drowsy while driving, in meetings, or
    while watching television?   Yes   No

Scoring: If you answer yes to three or more of these questions, you may be dealing with shift work disorder. Consult your doctor. He or she can help manage your symptoms. Only a change in shift work can resolve SWD, but there are some things you can do to minimize the condition, and they bear repeating:

- Avoid alcohol prior to bedtime. It will interfere with the quality of deep sleep.
- Get 7 to 8 hours of restful sleep each day.
- Eliminate noise and light from your bedroom.
- Try to stick to your sleep-and-wake schedule, even when you are off work.

NOT THE USUAL 9 TO 5: Other Health Effects of Shift Work

Conditions	Reason	Strategies
Cardiovascular	Shift workers have more adverse lifestyle behaviors, such as higher tendency to smoke, not exercise, and eat junk food—all of which hurt the heart. In one study, researchers compared 665 day workers with 659 shift workers. The shift workers had double the risk of low HDL cholesterol, 40% higher risk of high triglycerides, and 19% more fat around the waistline.	• Stop smoking • Exercise • Eat nutritiously
Breast Cancer	The risk may be associated with exposure to light during the night, when you should be sleeping. The hormone melatonin may play a role. This hormone is produced during the night but is disrupted by exposure to light. The resulting lack of melatonin may promote cancer.	• Don't take melatonin, unless specifically recommended by a physician. Supplemental melatonin may disrupt your body clock. It is better to let your body produce it naturally through normal sleep cycles.
Diabetes	Shift work can disrupt the body's insulin-making processes, potentially causing insulin resistance. With insulin resistance, the body doesn't use insulin properly. Glucose gets locked out of cells, and it clutters up the bloodstream.	• Have regular checkups to monitor changes in blood sugar. • Avoid refined carbohydrates, such as sweets, white bread, and baked goods. • Exercise on a regular basis to help the body better regulate blood sugar.

PART FIVE

....

Extra Help

16

Supplement Sense on the 17 Day Diet

I was checking out the kale in the produce section at my local supermarket when a patient tapped me on the shoulder and started a conversation with me about the pros and cons of dietary supplements. I was relieved that he found me among the fresh veggies, rather than filling my cart with gallons of ice cream.

We doctors give great, doable advice: Quit smoking, lose weight, ease up on sodium, wear sunscreen, and do skin checks for moles, but seldom do we talk about nutritional supplements. It's not because we don't believe in them, it's because we don't spend a great deal of time in med school studying nutrition. We spend most of our time pulling all-nighters, dissecting cadavers, studying pharmacology and which drugs are best to treat different diseases, and thinking about the first Mercedes or BMW we are going to buy after hearing we passed our finals.

Many people think we doctors don't like vitamins and other dietary supplements. This is a big misconception. We do like supplements. In fact, most doctors even take supplements and we recommend them to our patients.

There is a lot of proof, because researchers are very interested in doctor behavior. I have a couple of examples. The Council for Responsible Nutrition, a trade association for supplement makers, conducted an online survey in October 2007 of 900 physicians and 277 nurses. The survey asked these health professionals whether they took dietary supplements, and if they did, why? It also inquired as to whether they recommended dietary supplements to their patients.

The survey found that 72 percent of physicians and 89 percent of nurses in this sample took dietary supplements on a regular basis, occasionally, or seasonally. The main reason was for overall good health.

Now, did they ever recommend dietary supplements to their patients?

You betcha! Almost 80 percent of physicians and 82 percent of nurses said they did. This study was published in the *Nutrition Journal*.

In a more recent survey (2011), also reported in the *Nutrition Journal*, researchers surveyed medical specialists: cardiologists, dermatologists, and orthopedists. Over half the cardiologists said they took dietary supplements at least occasionally. So did 75 percent of dermatologists and 73 percent of orthopedists. Mostly, these docs took a multivitamin, although 20 percent admitted they used some herbal supplements. Seventy-two percent of cardiologists, 66 percent of dermatologists, and 91 percent of orthopedists definitely recommended dietary supplements to their patients. Cardiologists said they wanted to help their patients lower cholesterol. Dermatologists thought supplements would help improve skin, hair, and nails. And orthopedists recommended supplements to improve joint and bone health.

It is good news to me that so many doctors talk to their patients about supplements, because it is usually the other way around. Patients come to their visits armed with Internet information and studies about supplements and already have reached their own conclusions. Some even like to argue. There is so much information on the Internet about supplements that doctors feel outnumbered by online experts, most of whom do not have medical degrees. This is called medicine by Google, and it is overwhelming. Google "vitamin C" and you will get 44,000,000 hits. I will be a very old man by the time I've finished sorting out the conflicting opinions.

Nonetheless, I am constantly trying to keep up with the research on dietary supplements, because my patients, like the guy in the grocery story, want to know what I think. Some medical professionals argue that there are not enough studies of supplements. This is untrue. There are literally hundreds of studies each week reporting on the efficacy of supplements. The naysayers need to look at this research. Much of it shows positive results when the right supplements are used for the appropriate condition.

Obviously, it's important for doctors to know when and if a supplement is actually beneficial. By that, I mean the supplement can make a discernible difference in a patient's health. I pay attention to the supplement issue, because I want to know if I am helping or confusing patients.

Dietitians, who do study nutrition in college, say you can get all the vitamins and minerals you need from a proper diet. But the world is so complex, and food is so much less nutritious than it was a century ago, that there just isn't anybody who eats a good diet anymore.

So let's talk about supplements in general—what you might need for good health—and what specific supplements you might want to consider and talk to your doctor about in the area of weight control.

The Basics

While you're losing weight and exercising, your body has a heightened need for nutrition, and certain supplements provide a great backup. Vitally important to mention is that if you are considered very overweight or obese, well then, you definitely need nutritional supplements.

In 2012, a team of researchers at the University of Hohenheim in Stuttgart, Germany, looked into this issue by evaluating vitamin and mineral intake in 104 obese folks. Basically, the researchers found that the obese participants were low in vitamin D (which is important for weight loss), and several antioxidants, including vitamin C, selenium, zinc, beta-carotene, and lycopene. These people also had signs of inflammation in their bodies, as shown in elevated C-reactive protein. I think this study really underscores the need for supplementation, especially an antioxidant-containing formula.

Start with a multivitamin and mineral supplement, a once-a-day type, preferably an antioxidant formula. Like a lot of doctors, I recommend to adults that they take Flintstones vitamins—two a day. No more than that, or you'll find yourself trying to stop your car with your bare feet. I also like chewable vitamins, especially the ones that taste like Gummy Bears.

Men: Avoid supplements that contain iron because you don't need excess iron. It promotes cell deterioration. Women who are still menstruating may need iron.

I like to make sure people take multivitamins that contain folic acid and vitamin B6. The latter may lower the blood levels of *homocysteine*, a natural but not-so-good chemical believed to be a factor in heart disease. Folic acid is important for women of child-bearing years. Just 400 milligrams of folic acid daily can cut your risk of neural tube defects in your baby. Prenatal vitamins contain exactly what you need.

Specific Medical Conditions

It's true that certain supplements can help you if you suffer from a specific medical condition. Iron deficiency or anemia, for example, is common among women before menopause. If you think you may be suffering from anemia, you should talk to your family doctor, who will check this and recommend an appropriate iron supplement if required. Certain other medical conditions may also leave you in need of supplementation, for example, if you suffer from Crohn's disease, which reduces dietary absorption of nutrients, or a food intolerance that cuts out whole food groups. If so, talk to your doctor or dietitian. And if you are a vegetarian, vitamins B12, iron, and vitamin D can be difficult to come by, so you may need supplements.

To my women readers: No matter your age, it is a good idea to include calcium and vitamin D supplements in your supplement program. Both nutrients improve your bone health and cut your future odds of being afflicted with bone-crippling osteoporosis. I recommend at least 1,000 to 1,200 milligrams of calcium daily and Vitamin D, 800 to 1,000 international units (IU) a day. (For more information on vitamin D, see "Vitamin D.") If you are over 50, take 1,500 milligrams of calcium a day. And don't mistakenly believe that your multivitamin/mineral has enough calcium. It doesn't! If it did, the supplement would have to be as big as a horse pill. Your usual multivitamin has about 45 milligrams of calcium (8 ounces of milk are about 300 milligrams).

There are dietary supplements you can take instead of drugs to help lower your cholesterol, too. First, a heart-healthy diet can probably knock down your total cholesterol by 10 to 15 percent. Still, a lot of docs agree that your diet works most effectively in combination with cholesterol-reducing drugs, such as statins. I've see statins drop LDL and total cholesterol by as much as a third. They do this by helping to block the production of cholesterol by the liver. However, these drugs come with a slew of potential side effects. The most common side effect is muscle aches. Other complaints include migraines, nausea, fatigue, upset stomach, and muscle and joint pain. I see these problems all the time and, of course, they have to be managed.

Here's what I do for patients who can't tolerate statins but need to lower their cholesterol. I prescribe a combination of niacin (a B vitamin), fish oil, and flaxseed oil in these amounts:

- Niacin: 250 milligrams a day for two or more weeks until they experience no flushing, which is a common side effect of niacin. After two weeks, I increase their dose to 500 milligrams a day. Once they tolerate that dose well, I increase the dose again to 750 milligrams daily.
- Fish oil: 3 grams a day.
- Flaxseed oil: 1 tablespoon a day (this can be part of a salad dressing).

All three substances are natural supplements you can purchase at a health food store or your pharmacy. The combination works powerfully to lower cholesterol, but always check with your own physician before self-medicating with supplements.

Supplements for Weight Loss

As a doctor, I'm skeptical about any food supplement that people might believe is a miracle cure, especially for losing weight. A lot of people are looking for a magic pill that will burn off pounds without diet or exercise, but, of course, such a cure does not exist. There are a few supplements that can work with diet and exercise to help with weight control, however. Just keep in mind that your diet, along with regular workouts, is the only true cure.

You do not need any special supplements to help you lose weight on the 17 Day Diet. I want to make that clear from the outset. But if you want a little extra help (emphasis on the word *little*), here are a few with medical-journal research behind them, and not marketing hype.

Vitamin D

You may know vitamin D as the sunshine vitamin, because our skin makes it from interacting with sunlight for at least 10 minutes a day. An explosion of studies has found that most of us are deficient in vitamin D. One reason is that we spend less time in the sun, for fear of skin cancer, or we slather on sunscreen, which blocks not just harmful UV rays, but also the necessary interplay of skin and this vitamin. Because of the rush for the shade, we're getting less vitamin D in our bodies.

Another reason is that people are getting fatter. Fat holds on to vitamin D, making it less available to the rest of the body. Also, people don't eat a lot of dairy products much anymore, and dairy foods are fortified with vitamin D.

A vitamin D shortage is a risk factor for a host of other diseases, including cancer, osteoporosis, and diabetes, as well as circulatory and *autoimmune disorders*, in which the body attacks itself. Plus, vitamin D is very important for muscle strength. Research has found that bedridden patients quickly regain strength after taking vitamin D. I have concluded that vitamin D, and supplementation if you need it, is a rock star for building great health.

Lately, vitamin D has been the subject of a host of studies showing that it may help you lose weight while you're dieting. One study found that an adequate supply of vitamin D levels in the body at the start of a weight-loss diet can help people lose weight more successfully. The scientists assessed levels of vitamin D in the blood in 38 overweight men and women before and after they followed an 11-week diet. The men and women also had their body fat distribution measured with bone density scans. After supplementing with vitamin D, the dieters ended up losing almost a half a pound more, and they lost more fat from their bellies than anywhere else. The researchers noted, "Our results suggest the possibility that the addition of vitamin D to a reduced-calorie diet will lead to better weight loss."

A more recent study, this one conducted with women, found that supplementing with vitamin D (300 IUs a day) took inches off the waists of supplementers, but not in those who did not take the supplement. The women who lost belly fat were also taking about 1,000 milligrams of calcium, so the combination of the two nutrients may do the trick for trimming your waistline.

Before you dash off to the pharmacy for a bottle of vitamin D capsules, I suggest that you talk to your doctor about having a blood test for this vitamin. The test is for 25-hydroxyvitamin D. Normally, your doctor has to order a blood test, and some labs still insist that all tests be ordered by physicians. I think this is kind of dumb, but a lot of places (and doctors) like to be in control. I have never seen a convincing argument against patients ordering their own tests, especially if they can pay for them. These days you can do a lot of things—appear in court, buy stocks, sell a house—all without involving professionals like attorneys, stock brokers, or licensed real estate brokers. Why not be able to order your own test? Anyway, get the test. If you're deficient, taking a supplement at the recommended level will correct any deficiency.

How to take vitamin D: 800 to 1,000 IUs. Check with your doctor on correct dosages, if you're deficient in this nutrient.

Fish Oil

Fish oil does practically everything for you but your laundry. I mentioned it earlier as a way to help lower cholesterol (in conjunction with other nutrients) and, among other things, it helps you control body fat. This was first discovered in overweight rats. Now that we have a lot of thin, flat-bellied rats running around, scientists began to test fish oil in humans.

A 2007 study in the *American Journal of Clinical Nutrition* revealed that fish oil supplementation actually shrunk fat cells in overweight women. (We lose weight when fat cells shrink; fat cells never go away, they just get smaller when we diet and exercise.) The 27 women in the study supplemented with either 3 grams daily of fish oil, or a placebo of paraffin oil. (Yuck!) The study lasted two months. At the end, the researchers found that, in the women who took fish oil, the diameter of their fat cells decreased and so did levels of *triglycerides* (a dangerous type of blood fat). Naturally, the findings were positive; suggesting that supplementing with fish oil is a good idea for dieters. Other research has supported the weight-loss benefits of fish oil.

Supplementation with fish oil is especially important if you do not eat fish.

How to take fish oil: As mentioned previously, take 3 grams a day for good health and possible weight-control benefits.

The Arginine-Selenium Combo

Are you interested in having a flat stomach and smaller waistline? I thought so. And, if you're getting the idea that researchers like to study belly fat, you're correct. Anyway, listen to the results of a recently published study, and you'll be impressed. In 2012, Researchers at Urmia University of Medical Sciences in Urmia, Iran, assigned 84 post-menopausal women who had *central obesity* (an excess of belly fat) to one of four six-week diets: a reduced calorie diet; L-arginine (5 grams a day) and the reduced-calorie diet; selenium (200 micrograms a day) and the reduced-calorie diet; or L-arginine, selenium, and the reduced-calorie diet. In one way or another, all parts of these diets had positive effects. The supplemental arginine reduced waist size. The selenium helped the women's bodies regulate insulin. Insulin is a fat-forming hormone; when too elevated in the body, it contributes to central obesity. And, the reduced-calorie diet helped decrease triglycerides, a blood fat. What this means to you: Taking 5 grams a day of arginine and 200 micrograms a day of selenium could be beneficial to weight control.

That said, what are these nutrients and how do they work? Let's start with arginine. For background, *arginine* is an amino acid, one of 22 aminos that are the building blocks of protein. Arginine is the only building block for nitric oxide (NO), an important molecule in the body that helps with circulation. (Nitric oxide is not the same as nitrous oxide, or laughing gas.) NO regulates the tone and flexibility of your blood vessels, so it has an important influence on your heart health. Taking supplemental arginine may help boost NO levels, thus benefiting your heart and blood vessels.

Among the other little-known benefits of arginine are the following:

Hypertension. Arginine supplements may lower your blood pressure, according to a number of studies. That's because of NO's ability to relax and dilate blood vessels, making them more elastic and less pressure prone. Research does show that taking arginine leads to beneficial drops in systolic blood pressure and modest drops in diastolic blood pressure.

Immunity. NO is a key to immunity. White blood cells, which defend the body against invaders, use NO to decimate bacteria, fungi, and other nasty invaders.

Erectile Dysfunction. Got your attention, have I, guys (and girlfriends and wives)? Good. Arginine may be a natural Viagra. The same problems underlying blood vessel dysfunction also affect your ability to stay hard when you need to have an erection. Taking supplemental arginine has been shown to help the blood vessels of the penis dilate, and you know what that means: a better boner.

How to Take Arginine: If you want to try this amino acid for its flat-belly benefits (or other, ahem, benefits), take 5 grams daily.

Selenium

Selenium is an antioxidant mineral. I probably don't have enough space to write up this mineral's impressive—and long—résumé. Suffice to say, selenium is used to form antioxidant enzymes. These are powerful warriors against free radicals, and are involved in preventing cancer, heart disease, and arthritis.

As an antioxidant, selenium joins up with other members of the antioxidant family to help correct *insulin resistance*: the body's inability to use insulin properly to deliver glucose to cells for energy. Insulin resistance is involved in diabetes, metabolic syndrome, and obesity. In fact, people with full-blown diabetes have been found to be lacking in selenium.

You can get selenium from a number of dietary sources, mostly plant foods such as Brazil nuts, brown rice, and whole-wheat pasta. Meats and fish are also rich in selenium. Over the decades, modern farming practices have stripped the soil of selenium, so many folks just don't get enough from their diets anymore.

How to take selenium. It's wise to take 200 micrograms daily as a stand-alone supplement, or as part of your multiple vitamin and mineral tablet.

CLA

Clinical research on CLA (conjugated linoleic acid) began well over 15 years ago, and looked at whether it could burn fat and help develop muscle. Its first guinea pigs were not guinea pigs at all but, you guessed it: rats. Taking CLA did work really well, but of course you had to be a rat.

Let's fast forward a bit. In one weight-loss study, scientists discovered that when 134 healthy overweight adults took CLA for two years, it encouraged fat loss and possibly helped these folks keep their weight off. This research was published in the April 2005 *Journal of Nutrition*. There have been more studies like this one, so CLA does seem to have some benefit. However, as with any pill or supplement out there, you must take it in conjunction with a weight-loss diet and an exercise program.

A newer study emerged in 2012, this one from China, which was interesting to me, because I thought the Chinese were generally slim. Apparently not. Anyway, the researchers, who hailed from the Kaohsiung Veterans General Hospital in Taiwan, studied 63 overweight adults, who were given CLA or a placebo. The study looked at changes in body composition, mainly whether the supplement could trim belly fat. Well, it turned out that it could. The CLA takers dropped weight from their waist and improved their muscle-to-fat ratio, meaning that they developed muscle and lost fat. The study lasted 12 weeks and was reported in *Nutrition*.

When I review the research on CLA, it is almost as though researchers got bored with studying all its good effects on weight loss. Now they are studying its benefits in heart disease, diabetes, and the inhibition of tumor growth. Most of the results are turning out to be positive.

How to take CLA: Take 1 gram with breakfast, another with lunch, and another with dinner, for a total of 3 grams a day.

• • • • • • • •

There you have it—my recommendations for supplements. When you see me at the grocery store buying kale, now you can talk to me about other things like how the San Diego Chargers played or what the Kardashians did last week.

MISTER M.D., CAN YOU PLEASE TELL ME

Wouldn't It Just Be Easier to Prescribe Diet Pills for Weight Loss?

Drug companies are always racing to develop new weight-loss drugs, but they haven't had much luck. The Food and Drug Administration has approved only three drugs in the past 30 years for treating obesity, one of which—Redux—was yanked for safety reasons. I don't know what they did with the leftover pills. Maybe they were recycled into something a dieter could use, like exercise bands.

The drugs that remain—Xenical and Meridia—have been moderately successful. I'm not an advocate of popping pills for every little thing. Pills don't fully address the problem. By prescribing drugs instead of lifestyle changes, doctors ignore the unhealthy habits that have contributed to obesity. One of these diet pills, the so-called fat blocker, Xenical, the brand name of a drug called *orlistat*, must be accompanied by a low-calorie diet to reduce your weight by about 5 percent for most. Diets are vital, pills or no pills.

There's an ick factor with this particular drug. Fat isn't absorbed, so it has to go somewhere. And orlistat takers find out in a hurry just where. (Keep an extra pair of panties with you, or wear some diapers.)

Yes, some people's obesity is so out of hand that it might be dangerous, and I might prescribe one of these drugs.

About the only advice doctors can give is stop eating sweets, fat, butter, desserts, superburgers—basically, we want you to avoid anything the least bit tasty. We would make everyone do this if we could. Then we could stop worrying about the obesity epidemic and get back to other things like curing the common cold and filling out insurance forms.

Review

- Nutritional supplements can fill in gaps and provide extra insurance against any deficiencies.
- At the very basic level, take a daily multivitamin/mineral supplement.
- Talk to your doctor about supplementation: He or she may recommend calcium (if you're a woman), vitamin D, and fish oil.
- Though not a panacea or miracle weight-loss cure, some supplements may help with weight control. These include vitamin D, fish oil, an arginine-selenium combo, and CLA. These must be used in conjunction with the 17 Day Diet and a regular exercise program.

17

The 17 Minute Spot Reduction Workout

Kapow!!!

That's the sound of me blowing up a myth: spot reduction. Everyone has heard of spot reduction; everyone has heard it's a myth. Not so fast . . .

By spot reduction, I'm talking about the ability to lose fatty tissue from specific locations on the body, like from your thighs or belly, through exercise, and, to some extent, through diet, as I mentioned earlier. Experts used to think that spot reduction was impossible because, when you work out, your body taps into fat stores from every nook and cranny, not just from selected sites. However, in 2006, a study from the University of Denmark in Copenhagen turned prevailing scientific opinion upside down.

Researchers there took a group of guys and had them do leg extensions with a light weight on one leg only for 30 minutes straight. They did not exercise the other leg. Next, the researchers assessed blood flow to fat cells in both the exercised and resting legs, and they quantified the amount of fat released from fat cells in the legs.

Interesting: The exercised leg had a big surge in blood flow to it and a greater fat release, compared to the resting leg. So basically, the repetitive exercising for 30 minutes in one leg triggered the release of fat from that leg.

These results suggest that you can burn body fat selectively from the body part you're exercising; in other words, you can spot reduce. The study examined fat on the thighs, which is extremely fat-burn resistant, so it's good to see that by exercising, you can trim your thighs. Based on these findings, I think it's safe to assume that you'll get similar results in other areas of your body (like your tummy) from this sort of targeted, repetitive training.

The Danish study is not the only one to examine the spot-reduction issue. Scientists at the University of Connecticut gathered a group of 104 volunteers (45 men and 59 women), and had them do supervised resistance training in one arm only: their nondominant arm. Could exercise burn fat from the exercised arm? That's what the researchers wanted to know. The study lasted 12 weeks, and the researchers utilized MRIs to examine the subcutaneous fat in the trained and untrained arms.

At the end of the experimental period, in the men fat had shrunk in the exercised arm, but not in the unexercised arm, proving again that spot reduction is possible. As for the women, there was a smaller amount of fat loss in the trained arm. The scientists did not speculate on why the men lost more arm fat than the women. Nonetheless, I read this study as further evidence that you may be able to spot-reduce your body with the right exercise program. And that appears to be a repetitive resistance training routine with light weights, performed for a certain period of time.

Now, if you ask most exercise experts whether spot reduction is possible, I'm sure they'd say, "No way!" Show them this evidence, and they may reconsider their position. Spot reduction may just be entirely possible.

How This Workout Works

The 17 Minute Spot Reduction Workout applies these findings from the lab to the exercise floor. You'll work a typical trouble spot (tummy, thighs, and arms) for 17 minutes each day to spot-reduce and spot-tone those areas. You'll use light dumbbells and a resistance band and perform high repetitions with them. Women: Use dumbbells in the 5 to 10 pound range; men, dumbbells in the 15 to 30 pound range. Along with those two pieces of equipment, you need a watch, so that you can time your 17 minutes. You'll also do some cardio to help release fat from your entire body. I've laid out the workout for you here. Doing this workout six times a week (remember, each workout is only 17 minutes!), along with the 17 Day Diet, should help you get faster results and boot fat out of storage.

The Walking Factor, Cardio, and Spot Reduction

When it comes to cardio, we doctors prescribe walking for everything: weight loss . . . back problems . . . cardio rehab . . . depression . . . a fierce, stabbing pain in the wrist (only kidding, of course). In fact, we have been promoting all sorts of physical activity since time began, yes, even before Jane Fonda and Richard Simmons. The reason is that we understand the research: Walking and other forms of exercise have been shown to alleviate many physical and mental conditions, sometimes better than prescription drugs.

Quite often, I'll write "Walking 4X weekly" on my prescription pad if patients need to be less sedentary. This gets their attention. Science even agrees with me. In a Spanish study, published in the *Archives of Internal Medicine*, half the patients in a group of 4,000 were given general advice by their doctors to exercise; the other half got actual written prescriptions to exercise. Six months later, the patients who got the written prescriptions were more physically active than those who hadn't. Other similar studies have turned up similar results.

The way I see it, exercise is a form of treatment, maybe even the most important lifestyle pill you can take. Writing out a prescription for it just makes sense. If I just said, "Go home and exercise, and call me in the morning," my patients would be disappointed. They don't like going home empty-handed. So I write out a prescription for walking. The patient goes out of my office happy.

Now, back to the spot-reduction issue: Lately, I have learned that walking is a good spot reducer, mainly for the abs. With walking (and the right diet), you can shed abdominal fat more easily than fat elsewhere on your body. Cardio exercise like walking, jogging, or running boosts the output of the hormone adrenaline. One of its jobs is to increase fatty acids in the bloodstream, so that the body can use them for fuel. Fat cells in the abdominal area are very sensitive to adrenaline. In response to exercise, they liberate fatty acids quite readily. It's much easier to work off fat from the abs than it is from the thighs and hips, where fat cells are more stubborn.

While updating this book, I came across some fascinating research done by researchers at the Washington University School of Medicine in St. Louis, Missouri. They took men and women, aged 60 to 70, and put them on an exercise program for 9 to 12 months. The exercise involved walking or jogging for 45 minutes several times a week, on average (which is what I will want you to do). The results of this study were great: Everyone lost weight. But the really important outcome was that most of their weight was burned from their bellies.

It's not always best to rest your case on one study, so I dug a little deeper. I found a similar Canadian study that involved just very overweight women. They walked or jogged for 90 minutes, about four to five times a week. The study lasted 14 months. At the end of the study, the women underwent CT scans to see where they lost the most fat. Well, guess what? They lost more fat from their ab region than anywhere else on their bodies.

Based on this information, I've concluded that the best flab-busters for your midsection are cardio activities such as walking, jogging or running, or treadmill exercise. And that's good, from a doctor's perspective. Abdominal fat and visceral fat (which envelopes organs such as the stomach) is strongly associated with abnormal blood lipid levels, high blood pressure, and other cardiovascular risk factors. But when you drop pounds, particularly around your stomach, with those pounds goes these risk factors, due to various complicated biochemical mechanisms that would be too boring to go into here.

Walking helps prevent fat gain in the belly, too. One reason is that walking is a stress reliever. If you're under a lot of stress, the belly is like a landfill for fat. With undue and chronic stress, the stress hormone cortisol stays elevated and triggers surges in blood sugar. In defense, your body lowers blood sugar by disposing of it in the stomach. Walking, or any type of regular cardio, thus regulates cortisol, blood sugar, and weight.

Walking may be the best method of getting in shape and improving your health. It's easy to do, convenient, and inexpensive.

In addition, doing both cardio and resistance training through the week helps burn fat from all over the body, and is very effective at ridding the body of unhealthy visceral fat.

Getting Started on a Walking Program

If you're just starting a walking program, start out slowly the first week. Walk about 20 minutes three times a week, at a leisurely pace. Just move. For the next few weeks, increase your time to 30 minutes; again, just do it at a leisurely pace.

Listen to your body. As you feel more energetic, increase your time to 45 minutes. From there, walk four or five times a week. By this point, pick up the pace: Walk faster.

The next progression is to go for 60 minutes, four to five times weekly, at a pretty good clip. In fact, you may be close to jogging!

Here are some additional tips:

- Wear some sturdy exercise shoes designed for walking.
- Look straight ahead as you walk, and stay aware of your surroundings.
- Consider enlisting friends to walk with you, or form a neighborhood walking group.
- As you walk, flex your elbows by 90 degrees. Keep your arms close to your sides and swing them backward and forward as you walk. This helps burn more calories.
- Walk as briskly as your stamina dictates.
- Breathe naturally as you walk.
- Consider using a pedometer to log your walking miles. Shoot for 10,000 steps at the beginning of your walking program. Then try to overshoot that benchmark as you progress.
- Finally, consider enlisting your physician and other health care providers to walk with you and a group of your friends. In other words, start your own Walk with Your Doc program, like I established at my practice in San Diego.

The Exercises and the 17-Minute Workout Schedule

Monday:

Lower Body Fat Blast

Today, let's start remodeling your thighs and hips. We'll get the blood circulating to fatty areas and help metabolize and pry off that fat. Here are the exercises:

Dumbbell Squat

Grasp a weight in each hand; hold them alongside your body. Stand with your feet a comfortable distance apart. Lower your torso until your thighs are just lower than parallel to the floor. Return to the starting position, and repeat the exercise for 8½ minutes. Take short rest breaks if you need to. Try to keep constant tension on your thighs and buttocks as you perform this exercise.

Walking Dumbbell Lunges

These are an excellent shaping and toning exercise for your thighs and hips. For this exercise, you'll need to exercise in a large area such as a track or a spacious room. To begin, hold a dumbbell in each hand. Keep your arms straight and hold the weights at your sides. Step forward on your right leg with a large step. Lower your upper body until your right thigh is parallel to the floor. Do not let your right knee extend beyond your right toe. Your back left leg should be extended, but with a slight bend in the knee. Repeat this movement with your left leg, lunging forward, one leg right after another. Continue to step forward in this fashion for a full 8½ minutes. Take short breaks as needed.

You're done for today!

Tuesday

Belly-Fat Blast

Today, let's work on your belly fat with resistance training and walking. Let's annihilate some blubber with a few well-chosen exercises. Here's why I've chosen the first two:

In a study conducted to pinpoint the very best belly-flattening exercises, researchers at San Diego State University found that the two best exercises are the bicycle move and the reverse crunch performed on a chair. Both exercises beat out other popular ab exercises by a long shot, in terms of strengthening and isolating the abdominals. I've also included another of my favorites, the floor crunch.

The Bicycle Move

Lie on your back on an exercise mat or soft rug. Keep your lower back pressed as closely to the floor as you can. Clasp your hands lightly behind your head. Flex your knees so that they form 45 degree angle to the floor.

Lift your shoulders off the floor, bringing your opposite knee (left knee, for example) to your opposite elbow (right elbow, for example), while straightening out the other leg. Switch legs and elbows, performing the exercise in an alternating fashion. Repeat this movement in a controlled fashion for about 6 minutes. Do not do it quickly. Take short breaks (30 to 45 seconds), as your body dictates.

Seated Reverse Crunch
The other exercise deemed most effective in the research study mentioned above is the seated reverse crunch. Sit on a chair or a seated workout bench, close to its edge. Grasp the sides of the chair with your hands and lean backward slightly. Bend your knees and tuck them in toward your chest. Next, extend your legs straight out in front of you. That is the basic move: tuck/extend. Repeat the move for 6 minutes. Do not do this exercise quickly. Take short breaks (30 to 45 seconds), as your body dictates.

Floor Crunch
This exercise works the entire abdominal wall, while placing very little pressure on your lower back. Lie on your back on an exercise mat or soft rug. Bend your knees, with your feet flat on the floor. Clasp your hands lightly behind your head, and keep your elbows pointing outward. Bring your upper body and shoulders off the floor slightly, using the strength of your abdominal muscles. Return to the start position and repeat this move for about 5 minutes. Do not do this exercise quickly. Take short breaks (30 to 45 seconds), as your body dictates.

Tuesday: Cardio

Today, walk outdoors, on a track, or on a treadmill, for 30 to 60 minutes.
You're done for today!

Wednesday

The Arm Blast
Most men and women I know want to bare arms, but they're too embarrassed by the flab, especially at the back of their upper arms, otherwise known as the *triceps*. Here is a 17 minute routine to correct that. You'll need a resistance band to perform these exercises.

Biceps Curls

Drape the band on the floor in front of you and step on the middle. The wider you place your feet the more tension (resistance) you'll have in the band. Grasp the handles in each hand, palms pointed outward. Flex your elbows, and bring the handles up in an arc toward your chest. Keep your arms close to your sides. Lower slowly and repeat. Continue the exercise for 8½ minutes. Do not do it quickly. Take short breaks (30 to 45 seconds), as your body dictates.

Batwing Burn

When the backs of your arms get flabby and flappy, it's like you have batwings. So let's spot-reduce and spot-tone them with this resistance band exercise.

Wrap the band around a sturdy object such as a stair railing or immobile furniture. Face the point at which you secured the band and take a few steps back so that there is tension in the band (it should not be loose!). Grasp the handles in each hand and position your feet about shoulder-width apart. Keep your knees slightly bent. Bend over so that your upper body is just about parallel to the floor.

Flex your elbows so that your arms are at your waist. Press your arms back behind you until they are fully extended and your elbows are locked. You should really feel this in your triceps. Return to the start position. Continue pressing back and forth like this for 8½ minutes. Do not do it quickly. Take short breaks (30 to 45 seconds), as your body dictates.

Wednesday: Cardio

Today, walk outdoors, on a track, or on a treadmill, for 30 to 60 minutes.
    You're done for today!

Thursday

Repeat Monday's Workout.

Friday

Repeat Tuesday's Workout, including the walking routine.

Saturday

Repeat Wednesday's Workout, including the walking routine.

Sunday

Rest.

LEAN 17: 17 Exercise Technique Tips

Proper exercise technique is critical for reshaping your body. Here are some tips:

1. For this workout, use weights and resistances that feel relatively light to you.

2. After a couple of weeks, increase the weights and resistance, but they should still feel relatively light because you'll be doing many repetitions. By progressively increasing your weights from workout to workout, you challenge your muscles to strengthen.

3. Follow strict form as you exercise. Incorrect form reduces stress on the muscles and bones and can lead to injury.

4. Be careful to move only the joints and body parts specified for each exercise.

5. Take a firm grip on the dumbbells, so that you will not accidentally drop the weights. For standing exercises, distribute your weight equally on each leg. This will keep you from losing balance and possibly injuring yourself. Also, bend your knees slightly to protect your lower back.

6. To get the most from every repetition, lift the weight through a complete range of motion. *Range of motion* is the full path of an exercise, from extension to contraction and back again.

7. Perform the lifting and lowering motions in a slow, controlled fashion. That way, you'll better zero in on the muscles being worked. Fast, jerky repetitions, on the other hand, don't isolate muscles but instead place harmful stress on the joints, ligaments, and tendons. Not only is this an unproductive way to tone muscles, it's also a dangerous exercise habit to adopt because it increases your risk of injury.

8. Breathe properly. With every repetition, inhale just before the lift and exhale as you complete it. Try to synchronize inhalation and exhalation rhythmically with the motion of the rep. Do not hold your breath, ever; this can cause lightheadedness or even fainting.

9. Know your limits. Handling weights that are too heavy can lead to strains, a condition characterized by swelling and pain in muscles, and pulls, which are acute tears of muscle fibers. To avoid these injuries, increase your poundage gradually. Do not overdo.

10. Take rest breaks of 30 to 45 seconds if you need to.

11. Stay hydrated; keep a filled water bottle nearby.

12. Work out in a well-ventilated space if you are working out at home.

13. Wear comfortable, loose-fitting clothing.

14. Don't skip workouts.

15. After your workout, have a snack that includes a little protein and a little carbohydrate (like a smoothie). A snack like this feeds your muscles, which are hungry for protein and energy after workouts. By feeding your muscles within an hour of working out, you help them develop muscle tone more rapidly.

16. Record your progress in the *17 Day Diet Journal*. Jot down things like the weights you've lifted, the duration of your cardio sessions, how you feel, and other important progress markers.

17. Begin to see yourself as an exerciser and active person. Let this become part of the very fabric of your being.

As a doctor, I would rather see you lose weight through a good diet, exercise (because it is great medicine), and healthy lifestyle choices before committing you to a lifetime of drug treatment. Many people can avoid drugs with these choices, if they are given the chance. So, fall in love with an active, healthy lifestyle—doctor's orders!

Review

- Spot reduction is not really a myth. Fat burn to an area increases when you increase blood flow (through exercise) to that area.

- Not only can you spot-reduce, you can also spot condition specific areas of your body and change your shape for the better.

- Walking has been shown in various studies to help burn fat from the abdominal area.

- Combine walking with the spot-reducing exercises here, and you can begin to lose inches from troublesome areas of your body.

MISTER MISTER M.D.: CAN YOU PLEASE TELL ME

Can Exercise Ever Hurt You?

I get asked that question a lot by my patients; typically, it's asked by patients who, like the late Erma Bombeck, say things like, "Whenever I feel like exercising, I lie down."

Maybe you've heard some negative stories about exercise yourself. Someone keeling over from a heart attack while running. Breaking a leg on the ski slopes. A head injury while biking. A patient once told me that she gave up walking after getting a pebble in her exercise shoes.

There was one study, published in the *PLOS* medical journal, about this very issue. It was a review study that consolidated the results of several other studies, and it had doctors buzzing. The study said that in approximately 1 in 10 people, exercise could worsen cardio events, like blood pressure, triglycerides, or HDL (good) cholesterol. However, the researchers couldn't explain why. But to me, it's fairly obvious. If you have a medically diagnosed cardiac condition, you must talk to your physician about what sort of exercise program is appropriate. Actually, all of us should let our doctors know about our exercise program.

Science is funny in that you do need to read between the lines. And scientific studies tend to be conflicting at times. If you wait long enough, researchers will generate a new study that aligns with your wants and desires. As for me, I'm patiently waiting for proof that pizza cures the common cold.

But, as for exercise being bad for you? Nah. It lowers your risk for almost every serious disease.

17 OTHER WAYS TO SPOT-CONDITION YOUR BODY

After about a month, your body adjusts to the training load you place upon it, and you may plateau. The best remedy to prevent stalls is to change up your routine with other activities. Here are 17 to consider and how they work:

1. Sprinting for the lower body
2. Step sprints (sprinting up a flight of steps or bleachers two at a time and walking down) for the thighs
3. Cycling (stationary bike or regular bicycle) for the thighs
4. Spinning classes for the thighs and overall fat-burning
5. Running (up and down hilly terrain, if possible) for the thighs and lower body
6. Basketball for the lower body
7. Volleyball for the lower body
8. Touch football for the lower body
9. Soccer for the lower body
10. One-legged squats (while holding on to a sturdy object) for the hips and thighs
11. Zumba for the hips
12. Pilates for the abs and core
13. Yoga for the abs
14. Racquet sports for the upper arms.
15. Climbing, either rock or indoor, for the upper arms
16. Boxing for the upper arms
17. Martial arts for the upper arms

MISTER M.D., CAN YOU PLEASE TELL ME

When's The Best Time of Day to Exercise?

The short answer: The best time of day to work out is the time that works for you.

Luckily, some scientists have been working on this. But scientists are like judges on *American Idol*. They don't agree on anything, so their findings always conflict.

As for morning workouts, people burn 10 percent more fat calories by working out in the morning, one study shows. Bodybuilders, who are not scientists, swear by exercising in the morning before breakfast. They claim it is the best time to shed flab. Supposedly, after sleeping all night, your carb stores gradually deplete. Once you get up and get exercising, your body is forced to draw from your fat stores for fuel. But what do bodybuilders know? They only leave the gym for bodybuilding contests and more protein powder.

Most doctors will agree with me on the following: Do not try prebreakfast exercise under the following conditions: if you are a diabetic or suffer from low-blood sugar, because you could become dizzy or nauseated; if you are not much of a dawn's-early-light person and a morning workout sounds about as appealing as watching reruns of *Are You Smarter Than a 5th Grader?*

As for evening workouts, a recent study by a group of Italian scientists found that women who walked in the evening burned more fat than women who walked in the morning. It's not clear why, though.

Again, there's no bad time to exercise, except for maybe right now, when I'm hoping you're reading this chapter.

LEAN 17: 17 Ways to Burn More Calories Without Jogging

Activity and Effort Expended

1. Run errands. Walking briskly while lugging dry cleaning or groceries can burn about 120 calories in 30 minutes.

2. Fidget frequently. Research has shown that fidgeting, such as tapping toes and fussing with hands, blasts off up to 800 extra calories per day.

3. Get on top. Skip the passive missionary position and climb on top. This position decimates 4.5 calories per minute.

4. Take the stairs. Every minute you climb kills seven calories.

5. Take two. Taking the stairs two at a time burns 55 percent more calories than single stepping.

6. Rock out. Studies show that exercisers who tune in to music while exercising work out 25 percent longer.

7. Give your lover a massage. An hour-long massage burns 230 calories.

8. Have sex. An hour of passionate playtime kills 270 calories.

9. Pace periodically. You could burn about 100 extra calories during an eight-hour day if you walk around your office, pace while on your cell phone, or otherwise move around.

10. Kiss. Every minute you kiss someone you burns 1 calorie.

11. Don't order out. Cook at home. Spending an hour cooking burns about 150 calories. You can burn half of what you eat for dinner merely by cooking it yourself!

12. Sleep. You burn up to 200 calories while sleeping for about 7 hours.

13. Kick up your heels. Dancing burns 200 or more calories an hour, depending on the dance.

14. Do the hula hoop. This isn't just for kids anymore. In just 10 minutes, you can burn 44 calories. Plus, you tone your tummy while doing it.

15. Jump rope. Fifteen minutes of jumping rope burns 170 calories.

16. Play with your kids. A game of hopscotch can burn 222 calories over the course of 30 minutes.

17. Coach your kids' sports team. Coaching burns between 281 and 372 calories an hour.

BE A HUMAN PRETZEL AND KEEP WEIGHT OFF

The biggest challenge with managing your weight is keeping it off once you've lost it, wouldn't you agree? Now researchers are looking to yoga as one way to stay trim and fit. One study looked at folks in middle age, traditionally a tough time to keep weight off. It found that people who do yoga regularly gain less weight than those who don't practice yoga. Three cheers for yoga!

So, why does yoga work so well in this regard? Not because yoga is a calorie torcher (it's not), but because yoga seems to engender an appreciation of body and health in yoga enthusiasts. They eat less junk food, they don't binge, and they are less stressed out—all habits that help keep you at a normal healthy weight.

Source: *Alternative Therapies in Health and Medicine.*

18

The 17 Day Diet
Breakthrough Recipes

One healthy practice that will make a big difference in your weight loss is to cook your own food. Now, before you start to panic, rest assured that you don't need to shout and jump and spin knives, make meals that look like a major work of art, or get a degree from the Cordon Bleu. You need some easy recipes—that's all. I can help you with that.

This batch of recipes is easy to follow and simple to prepare. There are no long lists of ingredients, complicated cooking methods, or hard-to-understand directions. All the recipes are built around the foods you eat on the 17 Day Diet. Unless otherwise designated, the recipes can be used on Cycle 1. Many of the new recipes can be used on Cycles 2 to 4. Make sure you read the instructions as to when to use the recipe. And don't forget about *The 17 Day Diet Cookbook*. It is loaded with recipes and meal plans.

All the recipes here are low in fat and calories, made leaner and healthier by using cooking methods such as broiling, baking, or lightly stir-frying. When the recipes do call for oil, it is always a healthy one like olive oil.

Some of the recipes make just one serving. If others in your family are following the 17 Day Diet, you can easily multiply these single-serving recipes. Other recipes feature multiple servings. Any leftovers can be refrigerated or frozen. That way, you can defrost and/or reheat in the microwave for a quick, healthy meal.

Once you get the hang of this way of cooking and eating, expect to lose your taste for greasy, sugary stuff. Why? Because tastes are learned. Just as you learned to like fattening, sugary, or salty foods, your taste buds can be retrained to enjoy fresh, delicious, and healthy dishes. For example, it's possible to retrain your taste buds by using herbs and spices. Salt-free seasoning blends are a good way to help yourself get out of the habit of sprinkling salt on everything. Your taste buds do adapt to what you eat.

I encourage you to get creative beyond these recipes. Most of us use the same 10 to 12 recipes most of the time. Why not try tweaking them to fit the 17 Day Diet? Here are some suggestions:

- **Dairy Products.** If a recipe calls for high-fat dairy products, you can outsmart it. Substitute the low-fat or fat-free versions. For example, if a recipe requires one cup of regular sour cream, try using fat-free plain yogurt (Greek yogurt works great) in its place, or blended low-fat cottage cheese. Also, fat-free cream cheese and fat-free sour cream can be substituted; both taste like the original. Try mixing yogurt with low-fat mayonnaise in dishes such as coleslaw, and tuna and chicken salads. This is a great way to add more probiotics to your diet.

- **Meats.** When selecting ground meats, look for those 90 percent fat free or higher. Yes, they might cost more, but look at it this way: You are getting more meat for your buck, since you're not paying for all that slimy fat. And just to get every drop of fat out, drain excess fat after browning it. I am really obsessive about this. I put a piece of paper towel in a strainer and pour the browned meat in so the towel can soak up the fat. If a recipe calls for a high-fat meat such as bacon, you can reduce the fat by 50 to 60 percent by using real bacon bits or turkey bacon to impart the bacony flavor. Or try using Canadian bacon. It is lower in fat and calories.

- **Bad Fats.** You can reduce or eliminate fats in recipes. For example, when sautéing or frying, simply coat skillets and pans with vegetable cooking spray (0 calories) rather than using vegetable shortening or butter.

- **Spice It Up.** Get in the habit of using high-flavor ingredients, like fresh herbs, zesty spices, and seasonal fruit, to invigorate dishes, rather than gobs of fat or oil. Another tip: Buy an oil mister at a kitchen or housewares store (Misto is one popular brand). Simply pour oil, such as flaxseed or olive oil, into the spray bottle, then spray a fine mist of the oil over the pan or the food. This process cuts the amount of oil that you use drastically and cuts calories from fat.

- **Desserts.** Fruit makes a great dessert, but by itself may be boring to eat. Try dressing up a bowl of strawberries with a drizzle of sugar-free chocolate syrup. Also, you can easily redesign your favorite dessert recipes to yield less sugar, fat, and calories by switching to lower-fat ingredients and learning how to cook with sweeteners such as Truvia.

• **Salt.** Are you watching your sodium intake? If so, start by using half the amount called for in the recipe. Or try using a salt replacement such as Mrs. Dash. Another idea is to substitute lemon or lime juice, flavored vinegar, onion or garlic powder, pepper, chili powder, or other herb-only seasonings for the salt. Use low-sodium soy sauce or hot mustard sauce to replace regular soy sauce. Season food with spices and herbs as an alternative to adding salt.

Now—the 17 Day Diet recipes. Enjoy!

Dr. Mike's Power Cookie

⅓ cup unsweetened applesauce

2 tablespoons almond paste

1 tablespoon flaxseed oil

10 packets of Truvia

¼ cup agave nectar

1 large egg

½ teaspoon vanilla

¾ cup whole-wheat flour

½ teaspoon baking soda

1 teaspoon cinnamon

½ teaspoon salt

¼ teaspoon black pepper

½ cup vanilla whey powder

2 cups oats

1 cup dried cherries

½ cup sliced almonds

Vegetable cooking spray

Heat oven to 350 degrees. Beat together applesauce, almond paste, flaxseed oil, Truvia, and agave nectar. Beat in egg and vanilla. Mix well. Add flour, baking soda, cinnamon, salt, pepper, and whey powder. Beat thoroughly. Stir in oats, cherries, and almonds. Mix well. Drop the batter by large tablespoons onto a cookie sheet that has been sprayed with vegetable cooking spray. Divide dough so that you have 18 cookies. Flatten each cookie with the back of a spoon. Bake 16 to 18 minutes or until brown. Remove from oven. Cool and store in a plastic container. Each cookie supplies 128 calories and can be enjoyed on the Activate, Achieve, and Arrive Cycles for breakfast or as a snack. Each cookie counts as 1 protein and 1 natural starch. Use on Cycles 2 to 4.

Kefir Smoothie

1 cup unsweetened kefir

1 cup frozen unsweetened
   berries

1 tablespoon sugar-free fruit
   jam or 1 tablespoon agave
   nectar

1 tablespoon flaxseed oil

Place all ingredients in a blender and blend until smooth. Makes 1 large serving. Use on Cycles 1 to 4.

Yogurt Fruitshake

½ cup acidophilus milk

½ carton (3 oz.) sugar-free fruit-
   flavored yogurt

1 cup frozen unsweetened
   berries

Place all ingredients in a blender and blend until smooth. Makes 1 large serving. Use on Cycles 1 to 4.

Egg-White Veggie Frittata

Vegetable cooking spray

4 egg whites, beaten

1 Roma tomato, chopped

Handful fresh spinach

Salt and pepper, to taste

Coat a small frying pan with vegetable cooking spray. Add beaten egg whites. Stir in tomato and spinach. Cook on medium-low heat until egg whites are cooked through. Lift from pan with a spatula, and season lightly as desired. Makes 2 servings. Use on Cycles 1 to 4.

. . . .
Spanish Omelet

1 egg

2 egg whites

⅛ teaspoon salt

⅛ teaspoon black pepper

1 tablespoon olive oil

¼ cup diced tomato

2 tablespoons diced onion

2 tablespoons fat-free shredded
cheddar cheese

Combine egg, egg whites, salt, and black pepper in a medium bowl, and whisk until well blended. Add olive oil to a small skillet and swirl it a bit to coat the pan. Turn stove on to medium-high heat. Add the beaten egg mixture. As it starts to set, gently lift the sides of the omelet and let the rest of the egg mixture cook. Once the omelet is cooked throughout, place the tomato, onion, and fat-free shredded cheddar cheese over one half of the omelet. Carefully, fold the other side of the omelet over the fillings. Makes 1 serving. Use on Cycles 1 to 4.

. . . .
Mexican Huevos

Olive oil cooking spray

1 tablespoon chopped onion

¼ cup chopped tomato

½ jalapeño pepper, chopped

¼ teaspoon salt

2 egg whites

Spray a small skillet with olive oil cooking spray. Add the onion, and sauté over medium heat until transparent. Add the tomato, pepper, and salt, and sauté over medium heat for 5 minutes. Set the mixture aside.

Spray another small skillet with olive oil cooking spray. Add egg whites and scramble until done. Transfer the eggs to a plate and top with the tomato mixture.

Makes 1 serving. Use on Cycles 1 to 4.

Greek Egg Scramble

Vegetable cooking spray

4 egg whites

¾ cup chopped red onions

¼ cup diced tomato

2 tablespoons reduced-fat feta cheese

⅛ teaspoon salt

⅛ teaspoon black pepper

Combine all ingredients in a medium bowl, and whisk until well blended. Pour into a small frying pan that has been coated with vegetable cooking spray. Cook over medium-low heat until eggs are cooked through. Makes 1 serving. Use on Cycles 1 to 4.

South of the Border Scramble

Vegetable cooking spray

½ pound of reduced-fat Chorizo sausage or turkey sausage (remove the casings and crumble the sausage)

½ cup chopped green onion

4 grape tomatoes, sliced in half

1 small jalapeño pepper (2 to 3 inches), seeded and minced

4 eggs or 8 egg whites

4 low-carb tortillas

½ cup shredded reduced-fat Monterey Jack pepper cheese

Coat a large skillet liberally with vegetable cooking spray. Add sausage and sauté over medium-heat until well done. Add onion, tomatoes, and pepper and cook until vegetables are tender.

Whisk eggs in a small bowl. Add to sausage and vegetable mixture. Reduce the heat and cook until eggs are set.

Microwave tortillas for 30 to 45 seconds. Spoon mixture into the middle of each tortilla and top with shredded cheese. Roll up to form a burrito. Makes 4 servings. Use on Cycles 3 to 4.

Harvest French Toast

1 egg, well beaten

2 tablespoons canned pumpkin

1 tablespoon skim milk

1 teaspoon agave nectar

½ teaspoon vanilla extract

Pinch of pumpkin spice mix

1 slice whole-grain bread

Butter-flavored cooking spray

In a small bowl, whisk beaten egg, pumpkin, milk, agave, vanilla, and pumpkin spice until well blended. Dip the bread in this mixture until soaked through. Place the bread in a small skillet that has been sprayed with butter-flavored cooking spray. Fry on medium heat on both sides. Serve and drizzle with sugar-free maple syrup.

Makes 1 serving. Use on Cycles 2 to 4.

Blueberry Griddle Cakes

1 cup uncooked old-fashioned oats

2 tablespoons cornstarch

2 teaspoons baking powder

½ teaspoon cinnamon

2 teaspoons granulated Stevia or Truvia

1 cup unsweetened almond milk

½ teaspoon vanilla extract

1 egg

1 cup fresh blueberries

Vegetable cooking spray

Pulse the oats in a blender until they are flourlike in consistency. Add the cornstarch, baking powder, cinnamon, and Stevia. Pulse to mix.

Whisk the milk, vanilla extract, and egg in a medium bowl. Add the flour mixture, and stir well. Once thoroughly mixed, fold in the blueberries, until they are evenly distributed.

Spray a large skillet with vegetable cooking spray. Heat over medium heat. Once a drop of water sizzles on the skillet, you are ready for the pancakes.

Ladle a ¼ cup of batter for each pancake. Wait until bubbles form in middle and pancake is drying at the edges before flipping.

Flip and cook about 2 more minutes on the opposite side.

Makes 2 servings. Drizzle sugar-free maple syrup over each serving. Use on Cycles 2 to 4.

Breakfast Crisp

1 can sugar-free cream soda

2 apples, peeled and cut into wedges

1 cup uncooked rolled oats

2 teaspoons granulated Stevia or Truvia

1 teaspoon cinnamon

Butter-flavored cooking spray

Preheat oven to 350 degrees.

Place cream soda and apples in a medium saucepan. Heat on medium until apples are soft. Drain the apples.

Meanwhile, mix oats, Stevia, and cinnamon in a small bowl.

Coat two single-serve baking dishes with butter-flavored cooking spray. Add the apples evenly to each dish. Top the apples with the oat mixture. Spray the oat mixture with butter-flavored cooking spray until slightly moist,

Place the dishes in the oven. Bake for 30 minutes or until topping is slightly browned.

Makes 2 servings. Use on Cycles 2 to 4.

Salade Nicoise

½ to 1 cup cooked green beans, chilled

2 chopped scallions

1 small tomato, sliced

Lettuce (the darker, the better)

One 3-oz. can light tuna

1 tablespoon olive oil

2 tablespoons balsamic vinegar

Place cooked green beans, scallions, and tomato on a liberal bed of lettuce. Top with tuna. Drizzle with one tablespoon olive oil plus two tablespoons balsamic vinegar and season lightly. Makes 1 serving. Use on Cycles 1 to 4.

. . . .

Super Salad

Lettuce, any variety	2 hardboiled eggs, chopped
Cucumbers	2 tablespoons olive oil or flaxseed oil
Onions	
Tomatoes	4 tablespoons balsamic vinegar
Any salad vegetable from the 17 Day Diet lists	

Combine lettuce with salad veggies and hard-boiled eggs. Toss with olive oil or flaxseed oil and balsamic vinegar. Lightly season. Makes 1 serving. Use on Cycles 1 to 4.

. . . .

Balsamic Artichoke

4 fresh artichokes	Fat-free salad dressing
¼ cup balsamic vinegar	

Place artichokes in a large pot. Cover with water. Pour in balsamic vinegar. Cover and cook for approximately 1 hour over moderate heat, or until artichokes are tender, including the stem. Let cool. Serve with fat-free salad dressing for dipping. Makes 4 servings. Use on Cycles 1 to 4.

. . . .

Full-licious Salad

Two 15-ounce cans artichoke hearts, drained	½ teaspoon dried basil
½ cup chopped red onions	½ teaspoon salt, optional
½ cup chopped yellow bell pepper	½ to ¾ cup of nonfat Italian dressing
2 tablespoons salad olives, drained	Leaves of Boston lettuce

Combine everything but the lettuce leaves in a large salad bowl. Toss well. Arrange lettuce leaves on four plates. Spoon salad on top of lettuce. Makes 4 servings. Use on Cycles 1 to 4.

Crunchy Salad

2 cups thinly sliced cauliflower

½ green bell pepper, seeded and chopped

½ red bell pepper, seeded and chopped

3 green onions, chopped

1 teaspoon agave nectar

1 garlic clove, minced

½ teaspoon seasoned salt

⅛ teaspoon black pepper

½ cup fat-free Italian salad dressing

In a salad bowl, combine all ingredients except the salad dressing. Toss with the salad dressing. Cover and refrigerate for at least 4 hours. Makes 4 servings. Use on Cycles 1 to 4.

Southwest Slaw

One 11-ounce bag of Southwest chopped salad

½ 2.5-ounce bag of real bacon pieces

4 tablespoons salad olives

½ cup fat-free Catalina salad dressing

Mix the salad with the bacon bits and olives. Toss with the salad dressing. Makes 4 servings. Use on Cycles 1 to 4.

Asparagus Tarragon Salad

1 package frozen asparagus

¼ cup chopped green onions

2 tablespoons tarragon-flavored
  vinegar

2 tablespoons white wine

1½ teaspoons dried tarragon

4 tablespoons reduced-fat
  Italian salad dressing

4 lettuce leaves

Cook the asparagus according to package directions. Rinse with cold water and drain. Chill for 45 minutes to an hour.

In a small bowl, combine the onions, vinegar, wine, tarragon, and salad dressing.

Arrange lettuce leaves on individual salad plates. Place chilled asparagus atop the lettuce. Drizzle with the tarragon dressing. Makes 4 servings. Use on Cycles 1 to 4.

Cactus Salad

3 cups finely chopped paddles
  of nopal cactus, needles
  removed

2 teaspoons minced garlic

½ cup finely chopped red
  onion

6 finely diced Serrano peppers

4 diced Roma tomatoes

½ cup finely chopped cilantro

1 tablespoon olive oil

2 tablespoons white balsamic
  vinegar

½ teaspoon salt

Lettuce leaves

Place the chopped cactus paddles in a medium saucepan. Add enough water to cover the paddles. Add garlic and onion; cover and cook over medium heat for 10–15 minutes. Drain. Cool, then cover and chill about 3 hours, or overnight.

In a large bowl, combine the cactus, peppers, tomatoes, and cilantro. Toss with the olive oil, vinegar, and salt. Serve on plates lined with lettuce leaves. Makes 4 servings. Use on Cycles 1 to 4.

Spinach Salad

Baby spinach leaves (less bitter than regular spinach leaves)

Assortment of salad veggies (onions, cucumbers, tomatoes, etc.)

2 tablespoons reduced-fat crumbled feta cheese

1 tablespoon olive or flaxseed oil

2 tablespoons balsamic vinegar

Salt and pepper, to taste

Place a large bed of baby spinach leaves on a plate. Top spinach leaves with salad veggies and feta cheese. Drizzle with olive or flaxseed oil, mixed with balsamic vinegar. Season to taste. Makes 1 serving. Use on Cycles 1 to 4.

Marinated Vegetable Salad

4 cups raw vegetables (green beans, cauliflower, Brussels sprouts, artichoke hearts, etc.)

Fat-free Italian dressing

Lettuce leaves

Oil-free jarred red peppers

The night before, poach the raw vegetables in at least 2 cups of water until they're tender but still crisp. Drain. Place in a glass dish and pour fat-free Italian dressing over veggies. Refrigerate overnight. Drain and serve on a bed of lettuce, topped with red peppers. Makes 2 to 4 servings. Use on Cycles 1 to 4.

Taco Salad

1 pound lean ground turkey

1 envelope taco seasoning

Generous bed of lettuce

1 cup chopped tomatoes

2½ cups chopped onions

Salsa

⅓ cup shredded reduced-fat cheddar cheese

In a saucepan, brown the ground turkey over moderate heat. Add taco seasoning and cook according to package directions. Place generous servings of lettuce on 4 plates. Top with turkey mixture, tomatoes, onions, salsa, and cheese. Makes 4 servings. Use on Cycles 1 to 4.

Beef Fajita Salad

1 pound lean beef such as flank
    steak, cut into strips

Olive oil cooking spray

½ teaspoon of chili powder,
    ¼ teaspoon of cumin,
    ½ teaspoon of garlic
    powder, ½ teaspoon
    of black powder, and
    ¼ teaspoon of cayenne
    pepper, mixed

4 cups mixed greens

2 cups chopped onion

1 large tomato, diced

Chunky salsa

Spray the beef strips with olive oil cooking spray. Place the strips on a plate and season them with the spice combination.

In a large skillet, place the spiced beef strips and cook over medium heat until well browned.

In a large bowl, combine greens, onion, and tomato. Toss to combine. Divide the salad onto 4 plates. Top with beef strips. Top with salsa. Makes 4 servings. Use on Cycles 2 to 4.

Village Salad

2 tomatoes, chopped

½ teaspoon sea salt

¼ cup chopped red onions

1 teaspoon dried oregano

1 tablespoon olive oil

2 tablespoons reduced-fat feta
    cheese

Combine tomatoes with sea salt; let sit for 5 minutes. Mix tomato together with remaining ingredients. Makes 1 serving. Use on Cycles 1 to 4.

Lettuce Wraps

1 baked chicken breast, diced

1 scallion, diced

½ cup chopped red grapes

2 tablespoons chopped celery

1 tablespoon olive oil

Salt and pepper, to taste

2 to 3 Boston or iceberg lettuce leaves

Mix together all ingredients except lettuce leaves. Refrigerate until chilled. To serve, take 1 Boston or iceberg lettuce leaf at a time, and spoon a heaping tablespoon of the chicken mixture into the center. Wrap the lettuce around the filling. Makes 1 serving. Use on Cycles 1 to 4.

Spicy Yogurt Dip and Veggies

32 oz. fat-free plain yogurt

Garlic powder

Onion powder

Seasoned salt

Cut-up fresh veggies

Take a large metal kitchen strainer and line it with a coffee filter, white paper towel, or fine cheesecloth. Place the strainer over a bowl to catch the whey liquid that will drain from the yogurt. Spoon yogurt into the filter-lined strainer. Cover and refrigerate for 8 hours or overnight. In the morning, you will have a nicely thickened soft cheese (about 16 ounces). Season the cheese lightly with the seasonings suggested above, try your own favorite spice medley, or add freshly chopped herbs such as parsley, rosemary, chives, or thyme. One-half cup of yogurt cheese = 1 probiotic serving. Use as dip for fresh vegetables. Use on Cycles 1 to 4.

White Bean Hummus

One 16-ounce can white beans (drain but reserve ½ of the liquid)

2 tablespoons olive oil

1 tablespoon mashed garlic (from a jar)

1 tablespoon white wine

½ teaspoon salt

¼ teaspoon pepper

Cucumber, sliced

Place all ingredients except the cucumber in a blender or food processor and blend until smooth. Spread hummus on cucumber slices. Makes 4 servings. Use on Cycles 2 to 4.

Smoked Salmon Rolls

Two 4-ounce packages smoked salmon

4 tablespoons fat-free cream cheese

4 teaspoons capers

Cut salmon into 4 large strips. Spread each strip with 1 tablespoon cream cheese per strip. Top each with 1 teaspoon capers. Roll up each strip and fasten with a toothpick. Makes 2 servings. Use on Cycles 1 to 4.

Chicken-Vegetable Soup

1½ cups cabbage, chopped

1 large carrot, chopped

1 cup okra, sliced

1 large onion, chopped

2 large celery stalks with leaves, chopped

One 15-ounce can of crushed tomatoes

One 14-ounce can fat-free chicken broth

1½ teaspoons salt

¼ teaspoon pepper

4 baked chicken breasts, diced

Place all ingredients, except chicken, in a large pan and simmer for one hour or until vegetables are soft. Add chicken and heat thoroughly. Enjoy this soup for lunch or dinner. Makes 4 servings. Use on Cycles 1 to 4.

Greek Chicken Stew

2 boneless, skinless chicken breasts, cut into 1-inch pieces, trimmed of fat

1 box low-fat, reduced-sodium chicken broth

One 15-ounce can chickpeas, undrained

1 teaspoon minced garlic

Olive oil cooking spray

1 cup sliced carrots

½ cup chopped onion

Place the chicken pieces, broth, chickpeas, and garlic in a large saucepan and cook, covered, over medium heat for 20 minutes or until chicken is tender. Set aside.

Spray a small skillet with olive oil cooking spray. Add carrots and onion and sauté for 10 minutes over medium heat. Transfer to the saucepan. Cook, covered, for 30 minutes, over low heat. Makes 4 servings. Use on Cycles 2 to 4.

Onion-Leek Soup

1 tablespoon olive oil

¾ cup sliced yellow onions

¼ cup sliced red onions

½ cup sliced leeks, white part only

1 teaspoon minced garlic

2 tablespoons white wine

1½ teaspoons cornstarch

1¾ cups reduced-fat, sodium-free chicken broth

¼ teaspoon salt

¼ teaspoon black pepper

¼ teaspoon butter-flavored extract

4 tablespoons freshly grated Parmesan cheese

Heat the oil in a medium saucepan over medium heat and add onions. Cook until onions are browned and caramelized, about 8 minutes. Add leeks and garlic and cook until leeks are tender. Add wine and simmer for about 3 minutes. Add cornstarch and simmer for about 30 seconds, stirring. Add broth and bring to a boil. Reduce heat to low and simmer for 30 minutes. Add salt, pepper, and butter-flavored extract.

Ladle soup into four soup bowls and top each with 1 tablespoon of Parmesan cheese. Makes 4 servings. Use on Cycles 1 to 4.

Cream of Pumpkin Soup

Vegetable cooking spray

¼ cup finely chopped onion

1 teaspoon curry powder

1 tablespoon cornstarch, mixed with 3 tablespoons cold water

One 32-ounce box fat-free sodium-free chicken broth

2 cups canned pumpkin

2 teaspoons agave nectar

⅛ teaspoon nutmeg

⅛ teaspoon pepper

8 ounces fat-free cream cheese

Coat a skillet with the vegetable cooking spray. Sauté the onion until soft. Add the curry and cornstarch mixture. Whisk together. Add the chicken broth and stir well over medium heat. Stir in the pumpkin, agave nectar, nutmeg, and pepper. Bring the mixture to a simmer. Add the cream cheese and blend well. In batches, transfer the soup to your blender and puree. Place the soup in a large saucepan and heat thoroughly. Makes 4 servings. Use on Cycles 2 to 4.

Tortilla Soup

4 corn tortillas

Vegetable cooking spray

Pinch garlic salt

3 ripe tomatoes, chopped

2 cloves garlic, minced

½ onion, cut into chunks

1 medium Serrano chili, cored, seeded, and minced

6 cups fat-free chicken stock

2 tablespoons minced cilantro

Salt and freshly ground pepper

Preheat oven to 400 degrees. Spray each tortilla lightly with vegetable cooking spray. Sprinkle each with the garlic salt, then cut each into 6 wedges. Place the wedges on a cookie sheet that has been lightly coated with vegetable cooking spray. Bake the wedges until crisp, about 8 to 10 minutes. Remove from the oven and set aside.

Puree the tomatoes in a blender. Place the tomatoes, garlic, onion, chili, and chicken stock in a large saucepan or soup pot. Bring the mixture to a boil, then cook, covered, on low heat, for 45 minutes. Stir in cilantro, salt and pepper to taste.

Ladle the soup into 4 large bowls. Top each bowl with ¼ of the baked tortillas. Makes 4 large servings. Use on Cycles 3 to 4.

Stewed Zucchini

2 tablespoons olive oil

2 tablespoons finely chopped white onion

1 medium chopped tomato

1 chopped green bell pepper, seeds removed

4 medium zucchini, cut into ¼-inch cubes

2 teaspoons dried Italian seasoning

Heat the olive oil in a medium skillet. Add the onion and sauté until the onion is translucent. Add the tomato and green bell pepper. Cook over medium-high heat, and reduce to a saucelike consistency, about 5 minutes. Add the zucchini and seasoning, and cook for 5 minutes. Makes 4 servings. Use on Cycles 1 to 4.

Guiltless Potato Salad

2 pounds unpeeled small new
    potatoes, washed, and cut
    into wedges

One 32-ounce box fat-free,
    sodium-free chicken broth

4 green onions, finely chopped

½ 2.5-ounce bag real bacon
    pieces

½ cup fat-free Greek yogurt

1 tablespoon reduced-fat Italian
    salad dressing

2 teaspoons Dijon mustard

1 teaspoon seasoned salt

Place potatoes in a large saucepan and cover with chicken broth (and a little water if needed to cover the potatoes). Boil on medium heat until the potatoes are tender, about 30 minutes. Rinse under cold water and drain. Add onions and bacon pieces to the potatoes. Refrigerate until cold.

In a small bowl, whisk yogurt, salad dressing, mustard, and salt. Toss dressing with potato mixture. Refrigerate. Makes 6 servings. Use on Cycles 2 to 4.

Sweet Potato Apple Casserole

1 large sweet potato, peeled
    and sliced

2 Granny Smith apples, peeled,
    cored, and sliced

Butter-flavored cooking spray

¼ cup Nectresse sweetener

2 tablespoons agave syrup

½ teaspoon apple pie spice

Preheat oven to 400 degrees.

Layer the potatoes and apples in a small casserole dish that has been coated with cooking spray. Sprinkle each layer with the Nectresse, agave syrup, and spice. Spray with the cooking spray.

Bake for 40 minutes. After 20 minutes, stir the mixture to ensure even cooking. Increase the heat to 450 degrees after the first 40 minutes and cook for another 10 minutes. The casserole is done when the potatoes and apples are tender. Makes 4 servings. Use on Cycles 2 to 4.

Pasta Caesar Salad

One 12-ounce box whole-wheat penne pasta
¾ reduced fat Parmesan cheese
¾ cup light or fat-free Caesar salad dressing
¼ cup chopped onion
½ cup chopped red bell pepper
2 tablespoons chopped chives
1 teaspoon minced garlic
Black pepper, to taste

Cook pasta according to package directions. Rinse under cold water and drain. Let cool.

Add the remaining ingredients to the pasta and toss well. Chill. Makes eight ½ cup servings. Use on Cycles 2 to 4.

Brown Rice with Mushrooms

3 cups fat-free sodium-free chicken broth
1 cup brown rice, uncooked
Vegetable cooking spray
½ pound fresh mushrooms, sliced
4 strips turkey bacon, chopped
1 cup finely chopped celery
½ cup finely chopped onion
½ cup vegetable juice

In a saucepan, bring the broth to a boil and add rice. Simmer, covered, for 35 to 45 minutes, or until rice is tender.

In a skillet that has been coated with cooking spray, sauté the mushrooms until soft. Transfer the mushrooms to a small bowl or plate and set aside. Respray the skillet. Sauté the bacon, celery, and onion until they are tender (add a little water or extra broth if needed).

Combine the rice, mushrooms, vegetables, bacon, and vegetable juice in a casserole dish that has been sprayed with cooking spray. Makes 4 servings. Use on Cycles 2 to 4.

Picnic Beans

Three 15-ounce cans light red
    kidney beans, rinsed and
    drained

½ cup chopped onion

¾ cup reduced-sugar ketchup

¼ cup Frank's Wing Sauce

2 tablespoons Nectresse

1½ teaspoons liquid smoke

4 slices turkey bacon

Preheat oven to 350 degrees. In a mixing bowl, combine beans, onion,
ketchup, sauce, Nectresse, and liquid smoke. Pour into a glass baking
dish. Top with slices of turkey bacon. Bake for 45 minutes. Makes
6 servings. Use on Cycles 2 to 4.

Oven Roasted Veggies

Olive oil cooking spray

1 medium yellow squash, cut
    into slices

1 medium zucchini, cut into
    slices

1 medium yellow bell pepper,
    cut into ½ inch strips

1 small red onion, sliced

½ teaspoon dried oregano

¼ teaspoon dried thyme

⅛ teaspoon black pepper

Place the vegetables in a baking dish that has been coated with the
cooking spray. Sprinkle with spices and spray the mixture with the
cooking spray. Cover with aluminum foil and roast for about 20 minutes
at 375 degrees, or until tender. Makes 4 servings. Use on Cycles 1 to 4.

Salad in a Sandwich

½ cup alfalfa or broccoli sprouts

1 tablespoon finely chopped onion

½ teaspoon minced garlic

½ cup garbanzo beans, drained

1 tablespoon light Caesar salad dressing

2 slices fresh tomato

1 whole-wheat pita

In a small bowl, mix sprouts, onion, garlic, and beans. Toss with salad dressing. Place tomato slices inside pita and stuff the pocket with the beans-sprouts mixture. Makes 1 serving. Use this recipe on Cycles 3 to 4.

Meat and Bean Burritos

Vegetable cooking spray

1 pound lean ground turkey

½ cup chopped onions

1 teaspoon minced garlic

One 15-ounce can refried black beans

¼ cup chunky salsa, plus additional for serving

One 4-ounce can mild green chilies, drained

1 tablespoon chopped fresh jalapeño pepper, chopped

2 teaspoons chili powder

1 teaspoon cumin

Four 8-inch low-carb tortillas

Preheat oven to 300 degrees. Spray a large skillet lightly with vegetable cooking spray. Brown the turkey with the onions until turkey is no longer pink. Add garlic. Stir in the beans, salsa, chilies, jalapeños, chili powder, and cumin. Bring to a simmer, stirring frequently. Simmer about 20 minutes, or until mixture is thick.

Fill tortillas evenly with turkey and bean mixture. Roll up each one, tucking ends in. Place in a glass baking dish that has been sprayed lightly with vegetable cooking spray. Heat the burritos in the oven for 10 minutes, or until warm. Serve warm, topped with additional salsa, as desired. Makes 4 servings. Use on Cycles 3 to 4.

Eggplant Parmesan

1 large eggplant, peeled

4 egg whites

Fat-free Parmesan cheese

Vegetable cooking spray

Garlic powder, to taste

1 cup low-carb marinara sauce

Preheat oven to 400 degrees. Cut eggplant into ¼ inch slices. In a
shallow dish, beat egg whites and 4 tablespoons water until foamy.
Dip eggplant slices into egg whites, then into fat-free Parmesan cheese,
pressing cheese into eggplant. Place eggplant on prepared baking
sheet that has been sprayed with vegetable spray and sprinkle with
garlic powder. Spray vegetable cooking spray over eggplant slices. Bake
30 minutes, turning eggplant over after 20 minutes, until golden brown
and cooked through. Cover with 1 cup of low-carb marinara sauce.
Bake for 20 minutes, or until eggplant is piping hot and sauce is bubbly.
Makes 2 large servings. Use on Cycles 1 to 4.

Fried Fish

1 cup shredded wheat,
    crumbled very fine

2 tablespoons oat bran

½ teaspoon salt

½ teaspoon onion powder

½ teaspoon garlic powder

¼ teaspoon black pepper

4 egg whites, beaten

4 fillets white fish, such as cod
    or tilapia

Vegetable cooking spray

In a shallow bowl, mix shredded wheat, oat bran, and spices.

Preheat oven to 350 degrees. Place egg whites in a separate bowl. Dip
each fillet in egg whites, one at a time, turning the fillet so that it is well
coated. Dredge each fillet in wheat and bran mixture.

Arrange coated fillets in a baking dish that has been coated with
vegetable cooking spray. Spray each fillet with cooking spray.

Bake for 20 minutes, or until fish flakes easily with a fork. Makes
4 servings. Use on Cycles 3 to 4.

Ceviche

1 pound red snapper or sea bass fillets, cut into small cubes

1 cup freshly squeezed lime juice

4 finely diced tomatoes

½ cup chopped onion

¼ cup chopped cilantro

¼ cup reduced-sugar ketchup

2 teaspoons Tabasco sauce

2 teaspoons dried oregano

¼ teaspoon salt

Pinch freshly ground pepper

1 tablespoon finely chopped pickled chilies

Olive oil

Place the fish pieces in a glass dish; cover with the lime juice and marinate at room temperature for 2 hours.

Mix the tomatoes, onion, cilantro, ketchup, Tabasco, oregano, salt, pepper, and chilies in a medium bowl. Toss with the olive oil. Drain fish and toss in the tomato mixture. Makes 4 servings. Use on Cycles 1 to 4.

Sesame Fish

Vegetable cooking spray

1 pound tilapia

2 tablespoons olive oil

2 tablespoons rice vinegar

2 tablespoons light soy sauce

1 teaspoon chopped garlic

2 tablespoons sesame seeds

Heat broiler. Spray a broiler pan with vegetable cooking spray to prevent fish from sticking. Place tilapia on broiler pan. Whisk olive oil, rice vinegar, soy sauce, and garlic until well blended. Pour over fish. Sprinkle sesame seeds over fish. Broil at medium heat about 8 inches away from heat for about 20 minutes or until fish flakes easily with a fork. Makes 4 servings. Use on Cycles 1 to 4.

Salmon Burgers

1 pound skinless boneless
salmon fillet, cut into
1-inch pieces

2 egg whites, lightly beaten

3 tablespoons whole-wheat
bread crumbs

1 tablespoon fresh lemon juice

1 tablespoon Dijon mustard

¼ cup finely chopped onions

2 teaspoons dried dill

½ teaspoon salt

¼ teaspoon black pepper

Vegetable cooking spray

Place the salmon, egg whites, bread crumbs, lemon juice, and mustard in a
blender and pulse until well mixed. Transfer the salmon mixture to a bowl
and mix in the onions, dill, salt, and pepper. Form mixture into 4 patties.

In a large saucepan that has been sprayed with cooking spray, sauté
the patties until they are lightly browned on both sides.

Transfer the patties to a baking dish and bake at 400 degrees for
30 minutes or until cooked through. Makes 4 servings. Use on Cycles 3 to 4.

Elegant Poached Salmon with Dill Sauce

¾ cup fat-free, sodium-free
chicken broth

¾ cup white wine

1½ tablespoons lemon juice

1 bay leaf

4 sprigs fresh parsley

Two 6-ounce salmon fillets

¼ cup fat-free Greek yogurt

2 teaspoons dried dill weed

Seasoned salt, to taste

¼ teaspoon Dijon mustard

In a large skillet, combine the broth, wine, lemon juice, bay leaf, and
parsley. Bring the mixture to a boil. Add the salmon; make sure the fish
is covered by the poaching liquid. (If not, add additional equal parts of
broth and wine.) Lower the heat and simmer for about 10 minutes or
until the fish just flakes with a fork.

In a small bowl, whisk together the yogurt, dill, salt, and mustard.
Set aside.

With a slotted spoon, transfer the salmon to plates. Spoon the dill
mixture over each fillet. Makes 2 servings. Use on Cycles 1 to 4.

Salmon Lemonato

Vegetable cooking spray

2 pieces wild salmon

1 tablespoon olive oil

3 cloves fresh garlic, chopped

3 lemons

1 teaspoon dried oregano

Preheat oven to 350 degrees. Place salmon in a shallow glass dish that has been sprayed with vegetable cooking spray. Drizzle olive oil over the salmon. Top with garlic. Squeeze the juice of the lemons over the salmon and sprinkle with oregano. Bake for 25 minutes. Makes 2 servings. Use on Cycles 1 to 4.

Mexican-Style Shrimp

Vegetable cooking spray

¾ cup finely chopped onion

3 cloves garlic, minced

6 ripe tomatoes, chopped

½ teaspoon freshly ground pepper

2 bay leaves

2 teaspoons dried thyme

1 teaspoon salt

2 pounds uncooked shrimp, shelled and deveined

3 tablespoons chopped parsley

Coat a large skillet with vegetable cooking spray. Add the onion and garlic and sauté over medium heat until tender. Add the tomatoes and cook for an additional 5 minutes, while stirring. Add the pepper, bay leaves, thyme, and salt. Cover and cook over low heat for 5 minutes.

Coat another skillet with vegetable cooking spray. Lightly sauté the shrimp over medium heat. Transfer the shrimp to the tomato sauce and simmer for 3 to 4 minutes, or until the shrimp are fully cooked.

Serve on plates. Sprinkle each serving with chopped parsley. Makes 4 to 6 servings. Use on Cycles 2 to 4.

Garlic Shrimp

Butter-flavored cooking spray

½ cup finely chopped onion

2 teaspoons minced garlic

6 finely chopped Roma tomatoes

½ teaspoon black pepper

1 tablespoon dried Italian seasoning

½ teaspoon salt

1 pound fresh shrimp, shelled and deveined

2 tablespoons chopped fresh parsley

Spray a large saucepan with the cooking spray. Add the onion and garlic, and sauté until the onions are transparent. Add the tomatoes and cook over medium heat for 5 minutes, stirring constantly. Add the pepper, Italian seasoning, and salt. Cook, covered, over low heat for 5 minutes.

Coat another large skillet with the cooking spray. Add the shrimp and sauté lightly.

Add the shrimp to the tomato mixture, and simmer until the shrimp are cooked through. Divide the shrimp mixture among 4 plates and sprinkle with parsley. Makes 4 servings. Use on Cycles 2 to 4.

Shrimp Cocktail with Avocado Dressing

1 pound uncooked shrimp, shelled and deveined

2 cups bottled clam juice

2 large avocados, peeled and sliced

½ medium onion, chopped

1 clove garlic, minced

1 Serrano chili, seeds removed, chopped

2 tablespoons lime juice

In a saucepan, poach the shrimp in the clam juice, covered, for about 2 to 3 minutes over medium heat. After the shrimp are cooked, remove them from the saucepan, drain, and refrigerate.

While the shrimp are chilling, prepare the dressing by pureeing the remaining ingredients in a blender until smooth. Alternate layers of shrimp and dressing in parfait glasses. Refrigerate until ready to serve. Makes 4 servings. Use on Cycles 3 to 4.

Avocado Stuffed with Scallops

Vegetable cooking spray

1 pound bay or sea scallops

⅓ cup fresh lime juice

1 tablespoon minced fresh
oregano

1 tablespoon minced fresh
cilantro

Salt and pepper, to taste

3 large avocados, slightly firm

Serrano chili, minced

Coat a large skillet with vegetable cooking spray. Place the scallops in the pan and sauté 6 to 8 minutes on each side on medium-high heat or until brown and opaque. Remove from heat and set aside to cool.

In a bowl, combine the lime juice, oregano, and cilantro. Add scallops and season with salt and pepper to taste.

Cut each avocado in half, remove the pit and spoon out balls of the pulp with a melon scoop, reserving the shells. Gently toss the avocado balls with the scallops and spoon into the empty avocado shells. Sprinkle the minced Serrano chili on top. Makes 6 servings. Use on Cycles 3 to 4.

Bacon Wrapped Scallops

8 large sea scallops

1 teaspoon chili powder,
    ½ teaspoon onion powder,
    ½ teaspoon of garlic
    powder, and ¼ teaspoon
    cayenne pepper, mixed

8 slices turkey bacon

Vegetable cooking spray

½ cup agave-nectar based
    barbecue sauce

Preheat oven to 350 degrees.

Pat the scallops dry with a paper towel. Season with the spice mixture.

Wrap each scallop tightly with bacon and secure with a toothpick. Arrange the scallops on a baking sheet that has been sprayed with vegetable cooking spray.

Bake for 12 to 16 minutes, or until the scallops are opaque and the bacon is crisp. Remove toothpicks before serving. Drizzle barbecue sauce over scallops and serve. Makes 2 servings. Use on Cycles 2 to 4.

. . . .
General Slim's Chicken

½ cup cornstarch

½ cup cold water

2 teaspoons minced garlic

3 tablespoons agave nectar

2 tablespoons light soy sauce

½ teaspoon red-pepper flakes

3 large eggs, well beaten

2 boneless skinless chicken breasts, cut into 1-inch chunks

One 14-ounce bag frozen broccoli florets

Vegetable cooking spray

1 cup cooked rice, for serving

In a small bowl, whisk 1 tablespoon of cornstarch and water until very smooth. Add the garlic, agave, soy sauce, and red-pepper flakes; toss to combine, and set aside.

In separate bowl, whisk egg and remaining cornstarch. Add chicken, and toss to coat.

Boil broccoli over medium-high heat until just tender. Drain and set aside.

Spray a large nonstick skillet with vegetable cooking spray. Remove the chicken from the egg mixture and place in skillet. Over medium-high heat, sauté, turning occasionally, until golden, and cooked throughout.

Add the broccoli and stir.

Add the cornstarch mixture. Cook until sauce has thickened.

Serve with rice (½ cup per serving). Makes 2 servings. Use on Cycles 2 to 4.

. . . .
Chicken with Orange Sauce

4 skinless, boneless chicken breasts

2 teaspoons salt

½ teaspoon freshly ground black pepper

4 egg whites, beaten

½ cup oatmeal flour (prepared by processing ¾ to 1 cup of oatmeal into a fine flour)

Vegetable cooking spray

1 cup sugar-free orange marmalade

Preheat the oven to 400 degrees. Season the chicken with 1 teaspoon of salt and the pepper. Set aside.

Dip the chicken breasts, one by one, into the beaten egg whites. Coat well.

Spread the flour on a plate and gently dredge the chicken breasts in it, one by one.

Arrange the chicken in a single layer in a rectangular baking dish that has been coated lightly with vegetable cooking spray. Sprinkle the chicken with remaining salt (1 teaspoon). Spray each chicken breast with vegetable cooking spray.

Bake the chicken for 35 to 45 minutes or until chicken is tender and flour crust is brown. Remove from oven. Microwave the marmalade for 45 seconds or until syrupy. Serve the chicken and drizzle the marmalade over each serving. Makes 4 servings. Use on Cycles 2 to 4.

· ·

Oven Barbecued Chicken

Vegetable cooking spray

4 skinless boneless chicken
   breasts

¾ cup Frank's Wing Sauce

2 tablespoons Worcestershire
   sauce

1 tablespoon agave nectar

1 teaspoon chili powder

½ teaspoon dry mustard

Preheat oven to 350 degrees. Place chicken breasts in a baking pan that has been sprayed with vegetable cooking spray. Bake for 20 to 25 minutes. In the meantime, stir together Wing Sauce, Worcestershire sauce, agave nectar. chili powder, and dry mustard to make the barbecue sauce. Remove chicken breasts from oven and coat with sauce. Return to oven and bake for 10 more minutes. Makes 4 servings. Use on Cycles 1 to 4.

. . . .
Chicken Kiev

4 tablespoons fat-free cream
   cheese

2 tablespoons chopped fresh
   chives

2 tablespoons chopped fresh
   parsley

2 teaspoons minced garlic

½ teaspoon seasoned salt

4 skinless, boneless chicken
   breasts

1 egg, beaten

½ cup fat-free milk

4 slices whole-wheat bread,
   crumbed

Vegetable cooking spray

Preheat oven to 375 degrees. Mix together cream cheese, chives, parsley, garlic, and salt. Cover and freeze about 30 minutes.

Using a mallet, flatten each chicken breast with a mallet between sheets of plastic wrap. Divide cream cheese mixture into four equal pieces and place each on the center of a chicken breast. Fold up the chicken, and fasten with a toothpick.

Mix the egg and milk. Dip each chicken piece in the egg and milk mixture. Roll each chicken piece in the bread crumbs.

Place the chicken in a glass baking dish that has been sprayed with vegetable cooking spray. Liberally spray the chicken with the cooking spray.

Bake uncovered about 35 minutes to 45 minutes at 375 degrees or until chicken is no longer pink in center.

Makes 4 servings. Use on Cycles 3 to 4.

. . . .
Easy Gourmet Chicken

4 skinless, boneless chicken
   breasts

1 cup fat-free buttermilk

Vegetable cooking spray

½ teaspoon salt

¼ teaspoon pepper

2 tablespoons light soy sauce

2 teaspoons agave nectar

¼ cup orange juice

½ 12.75-ounce jar sugar-free
   apricot jam

Marinate the chicken breasts in the buttermilk, in the refrigerator, covered, overnight.

The next day, preheat the oven to 350 degrees. Drain the chicken. Place the breasts in a baking dish that has been coated with vegetable cooking spray. Sprinkle with salt and pepper. Bake at 350 degrees for 30 minutes.

While the chicken is in the oven, combine the soy sauce, agave nectar, juice, and jam in a small bowl. Pour this mixture over the chicken breasts and bake for 15 to 20 minutes. Makes 4 servings. Use on Cycles 3 to 4.

Turkey Black Bean Chili

1 pound lean ground turkey
2 cups black beans, drained
1 cup chopped onion
2 cups tomato sauce

1 tablespoon chili powder
1 teaspoon Kosher salt
½ teaspoon black pepper

In a saucepan, brown the ground turkey over moderate heat. Add the remainder of the ingredients. Simmer for 20 minutes. Makes 4 servings. Use on Cycles 2 to 4.

Old-Fashioned Beef Stew

1 pound red potatoes, peeled and quartered
1 large onion, quartered
2 garlic cloves, minced
2 cups baby carrots
4 stalks celery, chopped
1 cup sliced mushrooms

1 pound lean stewing beef, fat trimmed
1 teaspoon dried mixed Italian herbs
2 bay leaves
1 cup red wine
1 tablespoon Worcestershire sauce

Place potato quarters in the bottom of a large Crock-Pot, followed by other vegetables. Top with the beef. Sprinkle herbs and add bay leaf. Pour wine and Worcestershire sauce over meat and vegetables. Set Crock-

Pot on low and slow cook for 6 to 8 hours, or until meat is very tender. Makes 4 servings. Use on Cycles 2 to 4.

Catalina Grilled Steak

Four 5- or 6-ounce round, loin, or eye of the round filets, or any other lean cut

One 16-fluid-ounce bottle fat-free Catalina salad dressing

Place filets in a glass baking dish. Pour the bottle of dressing over the meat. Let marinate in the refrigerator overnight.

After marinating, grill steaks, basting with dressing frequently. Grill until meat reaches desired doneness. Makes 4 servings. Use on Cycles 2 to 4.

Drunken Pork Chops

1 cup Redd's Apple Ale or 1 cup sugar-free apple juice

1 tablespoon smoked paprika

1 tablespoon garlic powder

1 tablespoon sage

1 teaspoon dried oregano

4 thick cut boneless pork chops

Salt and pepper

In a large bowl, whisk together the ale, paprika, garlic powder, sage, and oregano. Pour into a Crock-Pot. Add the pork chops, and season to taste with salt and pepper. Cover, and cook on high for 4 hours. Makes 4 servings. Use on Cycles 2 to 4.

Apricot-Glazed Lamb Chops

⅓ cup sugar-free apricot jam

1 tablespoon raspberry vinegar

¼ teaspoon salt

½ teaspoon black pepper

4 loin lamb chops, fat trimmed

Preheat broiler. Combine apricot jam, vinegar, salt, and pepper in small saucepan; cook slowly, stirring, until jam has melted.

Place lamb chops on a broiling pan. Put pan in oven with the rack positioned closest to broiler heating element. Broil chops for 5 minutes. Spoon half of jam mixture over the chops. Broil 1 more minute. Turn the chops over and broil another 5 minutes. Spoon on the rest of the jam mixture and broil for another minute. Makes 4 servings. Use on Cycles 2 to 4.

Creamy Light Fettuccine Alfredo

4 cups whole-wheat fettuccine, uncooked

¼ cup Breakstone LiveActive cottage cheese

¼ cup plain non-fat Greek yogurt

¼ cup skim milk

½ cup fat-free grated white cheese, any type

2 teaspoons cornstarch

2 tablespoons cold water

½ teaspoon black pepper

In a large saucepan, cook the fettuccine according to the package directions, but do not use salt.

Drain the noodles. Return them to the saucepan. Add the cottage cheese, yogurt, skim milk, and ¼ cup of white grated cheese. Heat the mixture on low; stir well until everything is well blended.

In a small bowl, combine the cornstarch with 2 tablespoons of cold water and stir well. Add to the Alfredo sauce. Stir until the sauce has thickened slightly. Divide the fettuccine among 4 plates; sprinkle with the remaining cheese and the black pepper. Makes 4 servings. Use on Cycles 3 to 4.

Low-Carb Primavera Delight

1 spaghetti squash	2 diced garlic cloves
2 cups chopped fresh broccoli	1 tablespoon olive oil
1 small onion, diced	2 cups marinara sauce

Spaghetti squash is a great substitute for pasta. To prepare it, cut it in half (lengthwise). Scoop out the seeds and pulp as you would with any squash or pumpkin. Place it in a glass baking dish with about ½ inch of water, rind side up. Bake 40 to 45 minutes at 375 degrees. You can also microwave the squash for 8 to 10 minutes per half on high. Let the squash stand for a few minutes after baking or microwaving. Separate strands by running a fork through from stem to stern. Place strands in a separate bowl.

In a medium frying pan, sauté broccoli, onion, garlic, and oil until vegetables are crisp tender. Add squash and heat thoroughly. Serve on plates topped with heated marinara sauce. Makes 4 servings. Use on Cycles 1 to 4.

Mango Sorbet

6 cups of cubed, cored, and peeled ripe mango (about 4 pounds)	¾ cup light agave nectar
	¼ cup granulated Truvia
⅓ cup fresh lime juice, from about 3 limes	

Puree the mangoes and lime juice in a blender. Transfer to a glass bowl. Cover and refrigerate for 6 hours.

Remove the mango mixture from the refrigerator. Add the agave nectar and Truvia. Mix well. Refrigerate for 30 minutes.

Pour the mango mixture into the freezer can of an ice-cream freezer; follow the manufacturer's instructions for freezing. Transfer to a freezer-safe container; cover and freeze 8 hours. Let soften slightly prior to serving. Makes 6 servings. Use on Cycles 3 to 4.

Tropical Pistachio Pudding

1 package sugar-free instant pistachio pudding and pie filling

One 20-ounce can crushed pineapple in its own juice

One 6-ounce carton fat-free Greek yogurt

In a mixing bowl, combine pudding mix, undrained pineapple, and yogurt. Whisk together gently until the mixture is thickened and well blended. Cover and chill for at least 2 hours. Spoon into small bowls or parfait glasses and serve. Makes 6 servings. Use on Cycles 2 to 4.

Poached Pears and Oranges

2 tablespoons light agave nectar

2 tablespoons granulated Truvia

1 tablespoon fresh lemon juice

3 whole cloves

4 pears, peeled and cored, using a melon baller

2 small oranges

In a large saucepan, stir together agave, Truvia, lemon juice, cloves, and 2 cups of water. Put pears into the agave mixture and make sure the fruit is well coated. Bring the liquid to a boil. Reduce the heat to low; cover and simmer 20 minutes or until pears are tender when pierced with a knife. Transfer pears to a bowl. Meanwhile, peel oranges and trim off any white pith.

Add oranges to the poaching liquid. Bring it back to a boil. Reduce heat and simmer, uncovered, for 5 minutes.

Using a slotted spoon, transfer oranges to the bowl containing the pears. Bring the poaching liquid back to a boil. Reduce the heat to medium and cook for 10 minutes, uncovered, in order to reduce the liquid. Remove from heat; let the syrup cool slightly. Pour over the pears and oranges. Cover and refrigerate for at least 2 hours, or until chilled. Makes 4 servings. Use on Cycles 1 to 4.

Mom's Apple Pie

CRUST

1 cup ground almonds

3 tablespoons unsweetened applesauce

½ teaspoon granulated Truvia

½ teaspoon vanilla extract

Preheat oven to 350 degrees. In a medium bowl, mix together the ground almonds, applesauce, sweetener, and extract. Press firmly into bottom and up sides of a 9-inch pie plate. Bake 10 minutes until lightly browned.

FILLING

6 medium apples, peeled and grated

5 packets Truvia

6 tablespoons agave nectar

3 tablespoons oat flour

4 egg whites, beaten

2 teaspoons apple pie spice

Grate the apples on a box grater. Mix apples with the remaining ingredients. Pour over the baked crust. Bake the pie for 35 to 40 minutes at 350 degrees. Makes 6 servings. Use on Cycle 4.

Mint Choco Chip Soft Serve

1 cup fat-free Greek yogurt

2 tablespoons plus 1½ teaspoons Nectresse

2 teaspoons agave syrup

1 teaspoon vanilla extract

1 drop peppermint extract

2 drops green food coloring

⅓ cup sugar-free chocolate chips

In a medium bowl, blend all ingredients. Place the mixture in the freezer for 30 to 45 minutes. Transfer the mixture to an ice cream maker and prepare according to directions. I make single servings in a small ice cream maker, so this makes 1 serving. Feel free to double, triple, or quadruple the recipe for a larger ice cream maker. Use on Cycles 1 to 4.

Banana Ice Cream

1 ripe banana

3 tablespoons agave nectar

½ teaspoon vanilla extract

One 5-ounce can fat-free
   evaporated milk, chilled

¼ cup egg substitute

One 25-gram package of
   instant sugar-free, fat-free,
   banana cream pudding

In a small bowl, mash the banana until it is creamy. Add the agave,
vanilla, milk, and egg substitute. Blend this mixture well. Add pudding
mix. Blend well so that the mixture is the consistency of pudding. Place
in the freezer for 20 minutes.

Remove from freezer. Stir, then spoon into a single-serve ice
cream maker. Prepare following the manufacturer's directions. Within
10 minutes, you should have a delicious serving of homemade ice cream.
Makes 1 serving. (Double or triple if you have a larger ice cream maker.)
Use on Cycles 3 to 4.

Chocolate Candies

1 cup sugar-free chocolate
   frosting

24 sugar-free marshmallows

1 graham cracker, crushed

Spoon the cake frosting into a microwave-safe bowl. Microwave the
frosting on high for 2 minutes. One by one, dip the marshmallows
into the chocolate and sprinkle them with the graham cracker crumbs.
Place them on a plate. Refrigerate and serve. Makes 12 servings. Use on
Cycles 3 to 4.

Recipe Finder

Recipes for Cycle 1

Side Dishes

Entrees

Desserts

Recipes for Cycle 2

Breakfasts

Salads, Soups, and More

Side Dishes

Entrees

Desserts

Recipes for Cycle 3

Breakfasts

Side Dishes

Entrees

Recipes for Cycle 4

Desserts

19

Mister M.D., Can You Please Tell Me More?

The 17 Day Diet is simple, easy, and doable but, still, questions arise from time to time. Here are the questions I'm frequently asked, along with my answers. This information will help you.

Diet Issues

Q. *I just need to lose those last 10 pounds. How long should I stay on the diet?*

A. You should lose those 10 pounds rapidly on Cycle 1, if you follow it to the letter. Or you may have to continue into Cycle 2. It all depends on your individual metabolism. Everyone is different and loses weight at different rates. If you'd like to accelerate your weight loss and get to that goal faster, increase your exercise time and intensity each day. Just hang in there, don't get discouraged, and you'll achieve your goal weight in no time.

Q. *Can I switch some dinners to lunch, and lunch to dinners?*

A. Yes, you may switch lunches with dinners. It is a good idea to eat lightly in the evening anyway. I recommend switching lunches and dinners if you are a shift worker, especially. If you switch, be sure to not eat carbs past 2:00 p.m.

Q. *Is the 17 Day Diet safe for everyone?*

A. The diet is designed for people in normal health. Anyone who goes on this diet should have the blessing of his or her physician. Do not follow this diet if you have type 1 diabetes, any serious medical disease, or if you are pregnant or nursing.

Q. *I've gotten great results so far on Cycle 1. Can't I just stay on it?*

A. Congratulations! That tells me you are motivated to take care of yourself. Keep going! I don't advise staying on Cycle 1 more than 17 days, however. The diet is carefully designed to keep your metabolism charged up, to prevent plateaus, and to reintroduce foods gradually into your life. It's best that you follow all three cycles as described. Then after 51 days, you get to return to Cycle 1 for continued weight loss.

Q. *Can I drink fruit-flavored green tea on the diet?*

A. Yes, as long as it is not sweetened with added sugar. Many green teas in the supermarket are flavored with a hint of natural fruit and no added sugar. These are very tasty and can be enjoyed hot or cold.

Q. *When you say liberal amounts of a food, does that mean a huge piece of meat or second helpings of those foods?*

A. No. It's important to not overload your stomach. Use my Hunger/ Fullness Meter to keep that from happening. Eat until satisfied, not to the point at which you feel as though your stomach is going to explode.

Q. *There is a lot of protein on the 17 Day Diet? Why?*

A. Think of protein as construction material: the major component of all of your body's cells. It's responsible for building muscle and bone, creating antibodies, making hormones, and much more. For people who want to lose weight, protein is a top fat burner, and this is one of the main reasons the 17 Day Diet is higher in protein. Research studies over the past several years have found that protein helps you feel full and regulates your appetite so that you're not craving food all the time. Protein also forms your physique. Your body dismantles protein from food into nutrient particles called *amino acids* and incorporates them into new protein to build and rebuild tissue, including body-shaping muscle. And remember that the more muscle you have, the higher your metabolism, so protein is key for a healthy metabolic rate. Along those same lines, protein steps up the action of your thyroid gland, which is the master of metabolism. Research consistently shows that higher protein diets burn more fat than any other type of diet, so naturally I designed this diet to be protein rich.

Q. *I'm a vegetarian. Can I follow the 17 Day Diet?*

A. Yes. If you're a lacto-ovo-vegetarian, you limit your protein to dairy products and eggs. That means you'll obtain your protein from probiotics like yogurt, eggs, and beans and legumes (depending on which cycle you're on). Semi-vegetarians, who avoid red meat but eat fish or chicken, can easily follow the diet. Vegans avoid all animal proteins. If you're a vegan, you can still follow the diet. Simply use vegan meat substitutes at meals for protein and use a probiotic supplement in place of yogurt. The 17 Day Diet adapts to virtually any nutritional lifestyle.

Q. *I get bored with oatmeal and brown rice. What are some other whole grains I can try?*

A. There are plenty of other choices. Look into some of the so-called ancient or alternative grains: amaranth (high in protein), kamut (a cousin of wheat), quinoa (a seed), spelt (a relative of wheat), triticale (a cross between rye and wheat), barley (super-high in fiber), and bulgur (a delicious form of wheat). To find some of these more uncommon grains, you may need to shop at a big natural foods store or an ethnic food market.

Q. *Sometimes I can't eat all the food allowed on the 17 Day Diet. Will this interfere with my results?*

A. No, not at all. The 17 Day Diet is very filling. For many people, it's a challenge to eat all those fruits and vegetables for the first time. If you can't eat all the food, don't worry about it. Just don't substitute foods not on the diet for those foods.

Q. *I overindulged all weekend. What do you suggest?*

A. If you gained 3 to 5 pounds over the weekend, I advise that you go right back to Accelerate (Cycle 1) until you lose those pounds. After that, continue on with the other cycles to reach your goal weight. Or use The Transitional Day Fast to get back on track.

Nutrition Questions

Q. *Is it better to choose organic foods?*

A. These days, we need to find out where everything comes from and how it's been grown or raised. Is it organic, cage-free, free-range, or was it just grown in someone's backyard? We do need to reduce our exposure to toxins, or else they get stored in our body's fat cells. Scientists think this build-up of toxins may prevent weight loss. So, buy organic whenever you can. Eating organic foods helps you naturally rid your body of toxins. Organic food has not been treated with pesticides, either, which makes it a great choice for health.

Q. *You recommend a sweetener called* Truvia. *What is it?*

A. Truvia is made from the leaves of *stevia*, a plant that grows in South America and Asia. It is not really a sugar, nor is it a true artificial sweetener. Technically, it is considered an herb and is called natural zero-calorie sweetener. Truvia is formulated with *erythritol*, a sugar alcohol found in fruits. Both Truvia and stevia are more natural than some lab-produced artificial sweeteners, which is why I recommend them. You can also cook and bake with Truvia. Like anything else, use it in moderation.

Another sweetener to consider is Nectresse. It is made from monk fruit, a green melon that grows on vines on mountains in central Asia. Nectresse has zero calories, and you can bake with it.

Q. *Can I use other sugar substitutes on the 17 Day Diet?*

A. Artificial sweeteners are found in many foods these days, such as reduced-sugar yogurt, which is one of the recommended probiotics on the 17 Day Diet. All sugar substitutes on the market have been deemed safe by the FDA; we just don't know much about their long-term health effects.

There are a lot of artificial sweeteners out there. Among the most common are: aspartame (Equal), saccharine, acesulfame K, sucralose (Splenda), sugar alcohols, stevia (Truvia and Sweet Leaf), and Nectresse (made from the monk fruit). Unlike sugar, they are relatively calorie-free, and they don't kick up blood sugar. If you have diabetes, these are good choices for sweetening. Nor do these sweeteners promote tooth decay.

Sugar alcohols, such as mannitol and xylitol, are carbohydrates but not sugars, which make them sugar-free sweeteners. They are used in many diabetic products, because they are slowly absorbed and do not raise blood sugar to the extent that pure sugar does. They, too, are low calorie compared to natural sugar and do not promote tooth decay. Stevia is a newer artificial sweetener which is natural in the sense that it is not a chemical made in a lab. It is a natural extract from the stevia plant. So is Nectresse, made from a fruit.

My advice is to go easy on sugar substitutes and learn to enjoy the natural sweetness of fresh fruits.

Q. *I am trying to kick my sodium habit. Do you have any suggestions?*

A. You might start by using a light salt, such as Morton's Lite salt, to wean yourself off sodium. Start cooking with herbs and spices, too, especially garlic and onion powder.

When buying vegetables, purchase reduced-sodium versions. Look for sodium-free marinades for chicken, beef, pork, and seafood.

If you buy and cook with canned vegetables and beans, first rinse them under running water. This will remove as much as half the sodium.

The taste for salt is a learned habit. Just as you acquired a taste for salty foods, you can also learn to need less salt.

Q. *I've been hearing more and more about the health benefits of coffee and tea. But both have caffeine, right? Which has more?*

A. The fact that coffee and tea are good for you isn't new. The first written records of coffee, from about 1,000 years ago, mention it as a medicine. Over the years, herbalists have thought it could treat head and muscle aches, asthma and fatigue. Early references to tea in China involve boiling raw, wild tea leaves in water to soothe respiratory infections.

You already know that the caffeine in your morning cup of coffee keeps you alert and active. Now the *Harvard Nurses' Health Study*, a long-term examination of the habits of more than 100,000 nurses, has shown that there is a decreased risk of developing type 2 diabetes among participants who regularly drink coffee (caffeinated or decaf). Coffee is terrifically high in antioxidants, along with minerals, such as potassium and magnesium and B vitamins. All these nutrients might be the reason coffee guards against type 2 diabetes.

The good coffee news just keeps on coming: Research linked regular coffee consumption (three to four cups per day) to a decrease in the incidence of Parkinson's disease. Scientists have found that even an extra espresso may even help stave off mental decline as you age, according to a 2002 study published in the *American Journal of Epidemiology*.

So, grab a cup of coffee, sink into an oversized chair, and read the next question.

Q. *If coffee and tea are so good for us, should I drink more?*

A. Well, too much of any good thing becomes not such a good thing. How much you consume depends on your health and your caffeine tolerance. Most docs say that 3 to 4 8-ounce cups of caffeinated coffee or tea is the maximum that an individual should have daily.

Be aware that caffeine stimulates the central nervous and cardiovascular systems and is a diuretic. Too much coffee or tea can result in elevated blood pressure, insomnia, nervousness, or rapid, uncomfortable breathing. Also, tannins found in coffee and tea may decrease your ability to absorb iron. Drink your tea or coffee at least one hour before meals so you can digest the tannins before iron is released in your system.

Q. *Are trans fats in much of our food anymore?*

A. Fortunately, trans fats are going the way of the dinosaurs! These are a rather nasty, processed fat formed when unsaturated oils are hydrogenated. This process turns the oils solid at room temperature. Margarine and vegetable shortening are created like this and are good examples of trans fats. In cooking and food preparation, you need solid fat to achieve certain characteristics, like creating crispy crackers and flaky pie crusts. Solid fat also keeps foods from turning rancid.

Not all solid fats are trans fats though; some are saturated fats, including butter and cocoa butter, palm and coconut oils. But a while back, the food industry stopped using saturated fat because it was found to increase artery-clogging LDL (so-called lousy cholesterol) levels. The industry needed a substitute for saturated fat, so they unwittingly created a fat that turned out to be nastier than saturated fats, and trans fats were born. They seem to do funky things to cells, like distort them. We now know from research that trans fats raise LDL cholesterol, and they lower HDL (so-called good cholesterol), thus increasing your risk factors for heart disease. They also increase the risk of obesity.

If you're concerned about whether a food product contains trans fat, check the ingredients label for the phrase "partially hydrogenated." Partially hydrogenated oil means trans fat.

Q. *Is imitation crab allowed on the 17 Day Diet?*

A. Imitation crab is typically made from a whitefish called Alaskan pollock. The process involves grinding up the fish, from which the bones have been removed, mixing in fillers, tossing in a lot of salt, cooking it, and shaping it to resemble crabmeat. It is a good source of low-fat protein. Also, it is lower in cholesterol than true shellfish. Yes, you can eat it on the 17 Day Diet, but be careful if your doctor has told you to watch your sodium intake. Imitation crabmeat is really high in sodium, with nearly 700 milligrams of sodium in a three-ounce portion. That's almost a third of the sodium limit recommended for a whole day and almost half of the limit recommended for people with sodium-sensitive high blood pressure.

Imitation crabmeat tastes pretty good. But if you don't like to eat anything fake, or with ingredients that sound unnatural, stick to the real deal.

Q. *Every year I make resolutions to lose weight, and am successful, but after two weeks, I'm back to my old bad habits. How can I prevent those slips and maintain a healthy diet pattern for good?*

A. First of all, don't stop making resolutions. This is a good thing. Science says so: We know from studies that people who set goals (in other words, make resolutions) to quit smoking, lose weight, or work out regularly are much more likely to succeed than are people who don't make resolutions.

Second, take action. Sitting around, thinking about change, and talking about it doesn't make a difference. What produces change is action. Here are some actions you can take to prevent relapsing.

- Eat breakfast every morning and regular, planned meals throughout the day.

- Exercise regularly. This concept is really simple—move it *and* lose it.

- Guzzle more aqua. Water will really fill you up and assist in fat burning.

- Start a love affair with veggies. Supplement your meals with healthy salads and veggies and make your mom proud.

Health Issues

Q. *Just about everyone in my family is overweight. Is the deck stacked against me?*

A. Yes, there is the genetic piece to consider. People who research obesity discovered the blame-your-parents factor. Their studies involved fat twins who were adopted by separate thin families. The twins remained heavy despite their slim surroundings. The study concluded that the ring around your middle, or at least some portion of it, comes from your parents, not just from what you eat when nobody is looking.

So, yes, a family history of obesity may increase your odds of ending up overweight, but that just means you may have to put forth more effort than those without such genetics to get to a healthy weight. You can conquer genetics with exercise, too. In fact, researchers in Great Britain found that exercising can reduce the genetic tendency toward obesity by 40 percent. Their findings were reported in *PLOS Medicine* in 2010. You can choose to adopt healthy habits. We inherit predispositions to certain problems, including obesity, but we also have the power to decide what to do about them.

Q. *Does stress make people fat?*

A. It appears there is some connection, and it's based on the theory of the so-called caveman paunch. It has to do with where fat settles in the body, and it goes something like this. Guys get beer bellies for the same reason women get thunder thighs: It's a product of evolution. Cavewomen laid down stores of fat in their thighs and breasts to cope with the demands of pregnancy in the wild.

In cavemen, flight-or-fight energy was stored as belly fat. When cavemen went hunting and suddenly ended up being the hunted, their guts dispersed the fuel (fat) their muscles needed to high-tail it to safety. Since cavemen spent a lot of time fleeing, they never had much of a weight problem.

Nowadays, however, our predators are bosses, phone solicitors, and issuers of credit cards. They are irritating, and it's hard to get away from them. A good idea is to lace up your sneakers and go for a brisk walk. It's like hunting beasts but without any weapons. Regular exercise, seriously, really does prevent stress fat, plus a lot of other things.

Q. *I'm a smoker. I know I should quit. But I'm scared of the weight gain. What do you think?*

A. Let me ask you some questions: Are you sacrificing what might help your health in the name of keeping off a few pounds? Where is your common sense? You might be surprised to learn that if you exercise while quitting smoking, you won't gain weight.

Kicking butt with exercise will help you kick your cigarette habit. An Austrian study turned up a successful program for quitting smoking that involved exercise. They put a group of smokers on an exercise regimen that involved a combo of cardio and strength training. The smokers also used a nicotine replacement method of their choice, such as a patch, gum, inhaler, or a combination of these. One group exercised; the other did not. After three months, 80 percent of the exercising smokers turned into ex-smokers, while only 52 percent of those who used nicotine replacement alone (no exercising) had stopped smoking. What these results tell me is that exercise may be one of the top tools we have for getting people to quit. I feel that once smokers get that endorphin high from exercise, and start breathing better because of exercise, they just don't want to smoke anymore. If you haven't yet used exercise in your attempt-to-quit efforts, learn a lesson from this research: get moving!

Q. *I'm 56, and my doctor told me I have prediabetes. Which tests do I need? How can I prevent diabetes?*

A. *Prediabetes* means that your blood sugar levels are abnormally high, but not high enough to be diagnosed with full-blown diabetes. However, if you are prediabetic, you have a substantially increased chance of heart attack, stroke, cancer, kidney disease, blindness, nerve damage, and several other serious conditions.

Because you've been diagnosed with prediabetes, your doctor may recommend you check your blood sugar at home. There are some relatively easy, pain-free ways to do this, and you can get the kits at your pharmacy. In addition, your doc will order some specific tests for you to have annually. The two most important are the fasting blood glucose test, and the hemoglobin A1C (HgbA1C). With the fasting blood glucose test, you will be asked to fast overnight. Your blood will be drawn at a lab the next day and analyzed. Normal blood glucose levels are less than 100 milligrams per deciliter (mg/dl). The Hemoglobin A1C (HgbA1C) Is also a blood test. It averages any blood sugar elevations during a previous three-month period. A normal value for the HgbAlC is from 4 to 6 percent, and the goal for those with diabetes is to get below seven percent. Have your HgbA1C checked at least twice a year, more often if your doctor recommends it.

There are several things you can do to help treat prediabetes and prevent the onset of type 2:

- **Eat a healthy diet and take off weight:** Losing only 5 percent to 7 percent of your current body weight can usually bring your blood sugar to normal ranges.

- **Exercise:** At the very minimum, shoot for at least 30 minutes of activity a day, 5 days per week. Body fat prevents the ability of insulin ability to lower blood sugar. With less fat on your body, your blood sugar can normalize.

- **Treat high blood pressure and cholesterol:** If you have been told that you have either of these conditions, speak to your doctor on the best course of treatment to get them in check.

- **Quit smoking:** Diabetes is not the only reason to quit, as smoking contributes to many other health problems.

- **Educate yourself:** Education is key for prediabetes and type 2 diabetes management. Diabetes is a complex condition and needs close monitoring to help you remain as active and healthy as possible. Most insurance plans provide coverage for diabetes education programs, and they are very helpful in assisting newly diagnosed patients with diabetes management.

Q. *What are the best foods for my joints?*

A. If your joints hurt, they might be inflamed. But popping painkillers isn't the only way to stop the pain. Eating a fresh, unprocessed diet, as I suggest on the 17 Day Diet, can help alleviate the pain, too. Try eating high-omega-3 fish like sardines, wild salmon, or cod at least twice per week. Omega-3 fatty acids keep your joints in good shape and may even help arthritic joints. For protecting cells against inflammation, enjoy daily servings of vitamin-rich and mineral-rich whole grains and legumes, fruits (particularly berries), and vegetables—basically all the foods that are a part of the 17 Day Diet Another common yet generally safe remedy is glucosamine, available as a supplement. Many people get relief from taking it. Consult your doctor about whether to take it, which kind to take, and how much.

Q. *My HDL cholesterol is low. What can I do to raise it?*

A. Losing weight and working out regularly are two effective ways to elevate your good HDL cholesterol. This is one cholesterol number that you want to be high (the others should be low). If your HDL is 60 or above, you have a lower risk of heart disease. If your HDL is 40 or below, you have a higher risk. Incidentally, people with low HDL levels are often overweight, particularly around the tummy. This means there is a strong connection between weight and HDL levels.

If you can get to your goal weight and stay there, you can raise your HDL levels anywhere from 5 to 20 percent, according to research. Some of the best activities to raise HDL are swimming and walking. I've seen folks in my Walk with Your Doc group who have changed their HDL levels as a result of walking. As for diet, eat heart-healthy fats like olive oil and fish oil in moderate amounts; both are beneficial to HDL. There are other lifestyle measures you can take too: stop smoking if you smoke (smoking lowers HDL) and keep your blood sugar under control.

Genetics play a role in your HDL levels, and it's hard to change genetics. But with diet, exercise, and lifestyle changes you have the breakthrough tools to help you do it. All of these are the best medicine, plus, they're safe, effective, and cheap.

Q. *Which foods should I eat to improve my skin?*

A. One of the pieces of feedback I have received over the past few years is the effect the diet has on skin. People are noticeably glowing, as seen in their skin health. The foods on the diet are truly beauty foods. For example: Salmon is an excellent source of omega-3 fatty acids, which moisturize your skin from within. Kiwis, citrus fruits, blueberries, and bell peppers bestow the skin with vitamin C, which helps prevent wrinkles. Oysters are rich in zinc, crucial for collagen production (*collagen* is a protein that makes skin firm). Think of sweet potatoes and tomatoes as nutrient sunscreens. They contain beneficial chemicals called carotenoids that protect skin against damaging UV rays.

Q. *I've heard that being overweight is a risk factor for cancer. Does losing weight reduce risk?*

A. Research estimates that overweight and obesity in the U.S. account for 14 percent of cancer deaths among men and 20 percent among women. So, it would seem that losing weight would help, although scientists can't yet say for sure.

We do know this, however: Getting rid of excess body fat can regulate and normalize insulin, insulin-related growth factors, and certain hormones, like estrogen. All these compounds can accelerate the process of cancer development. Each loss or gain of excess body fat seems to lower cancer risk.

Q. *Does sugar feed cancer?*

A. All the cells in the body use sugar (glucose) for fuel, and research does suggest that cancer cells gobble up blood sugar more quickly than healthy cells do. Plus, high blood sugar causes the body to churn out excess insulin; this excess may promote the growth of cancer cells.

I know this sounds scary, but it doesn't mean you have to avoid all sugar-containing foods. Of course, it is not a great idea to eat a lot of sugar anyway, but at least curtail it. One of the best ways to prevent cancer is to stick to natural foods: healthful vegetables, fruits, whole grains, and low-fat dairy sources. Other preventive measures include weight control, regular exercise, a high-fiber diet, and avoidance of toxins and environmental pollutants.

Food Allergies and Intolerances

Q. *An allergist told me recently I suffer from lactose intolerance. How can I adjust my lifestyle accordingly?*

A. Lactose intolerance is caused by a lack of one or more enzymes that digest lactose, the carbohydrate in milk. Symptoms are bloating, diarrhea, gas, nausea, and abdominal cramps. Unfortunately, the recommended treatment is a lactose-free diet. If you avoid all dairy products you should also take calcium supplements. You can also buy lactose drops or tablets which can sometimes help you digest dairy products, if taken before eating them. If you're lactose intolerant, you'll likely find yogurt much easier on your tummy than milk. The friendly bacteria in yogurt feast upon its lactose, so there is less to disturb you. You shouldn't have any trouble following the 17 Day Diet with this food sensitivity.

Q. *I have to be on a gluten-free diet. What are some gluten-free foods?*

A. For background, about 1 out of 133 people in the United States has *celiac disease*, an autoimmune intestinal disorder that causes severe adverse reactions to proteins found in wheat and related grains. Even more people are intolerant to gluten. For people with severe allergies to gluten, it's the difference between life and death, and a gluten-free diet is the only means of treatment. It prevents the complications of untreated celiac disease, such as osteoporosis, anemia, and certain forms of cancer. For people with intolerances to gluten, the benefits of a gluten-free diet are many: fewer sinus infections, more energy, less brain fog, or less gastrointestinal upset. Some people lose weight on a gluten-free diet, but that may be because many high-calorie foods contain wheat, which is a carbohydrate.

Here is partial list of gluten-free foods:

- Milk (nonfat dry milk)
- 100 percent vegetable juices

- Fresh fruits and vegetables that are not coated with a wax or resin that contains gluten
- A variety of single-ingredient foods: eggs, lentils, seeds like flax, tree nuts like almonds, no gluten-containing grains like corn, meats, fresh fish, and fresh shellfish
- Gluten-free foods such as bread, pastas, and special cereals

Foods that are not gluten-free include:

- Barley, common wheat, rye, spelt, kamut, triticale
- Farina, vital gluten, semolina, malt vinegar

As for oatmeal, no one agrees yet whether people with celiac disease can eat it. To be on the safe side, purchase gluten-free oatmeal if you're an oat lover.

By the way, if you're on a gluten-free diet, you can easily follow the 17 Day Diet by making food substitutions to include gluten-free products.

• • • • • • • •

Keep those cards and letters coming . . . and visit me on the 17 Day website, www.the17daydiet.com, for more help and advice on how to live the diet and stay healthy and fit.

REFERENCES

Much of the material in this book comes from computer searches of medical databases of abstracts, medical news reports, and health articles in both popular and specialized publications, as well as scientific reports in peer-reviewed journals.

Chapter 1: Just Give Me 17 Days

Binks, M. 2005. Duke study reports sex, self-esteem diminish for morbidly obese. *CDS Review* 98(4):28–29.

Bui, C., 2010. Acute effect of a single high-fat meal on forearm blood flow, blood pressure and heart rate in healthy male Asians and Caucasians: a pilot study. *The Southeast Asia Journal of Tropical Health and Public Health* 41:490–500.

Claessens, M., et al. 2009. The effect of a low-fat, high-protein or high-carbohydrate ad libitum diet on weight loss maintenance and metabolic risk factors. *International Journal of Obesity* 33:296–304.

Gunn, D. A. 2009. Why some women look young for their age. *PLOS One* 4:e8021.

Hanninen, O., et al. 1992. Effects of eating an uncooked vegetable diet for one week. *Appetite* 19:243–254.

Henkin, Y., and Shai, I. 2003. Dietary treatment of hypercholesterolemia: can we predict long-term success? *Journal of the American College of Nutrition* 22:555–561.

Janiszewski, P. M., and Ross, R. 2010. Effects of weight loss among metabolically healthy obese men and women. *Diabetes Care* 33:1957–1959.

Jenkins, D. J., et al. 2009. The effect of a plant-based low-carbohydrate ("Eco-Atkins") diet on body weight and blood lipid concentrations in hyperlipidemic subjects. *Archives of Internal Medicine* 169:1046–1054.

Johnston, C. S., 2002. Postprandial thermogenesis is increased 100% on a high-protein, low-fat diet versus a high-carbohydrate, low-fat diet in healthy, young women. *Journal of the American College of Nutrition* 21:55–61.

Kiortsis, D. N., et al. 2001 Changes in lipoprotein(a) levels and hormonal correlations during a weight reduction program. *Nutrition, Metabolism, and Cardiovascular Diseases* 11:153–157.

Laaksonen D. E., et al. 2003. Relationships between changes in abdominal fat distribution and insulin sensitivity during a very low calorie diet in abdominally obese men and women. *Nutrition, Metabolism, and Cardiovascular Diseases* 13:349–356.

Lapidus, L. 1984. Distribution of adipose tissue and risk of cardiovascular disease and death: a 12–year follow-up of participants in the population study of women in Gothenburg, Sweden. *British Medical Journal* 289:1257.

Leigh, Gibson E., and Green, M.W. 2002. Nutritional influences on cognitive function: mechanisms of susceptibility. *Nutrition Research Reviews* 15:169–206.

Maconochie, N. 2007. Risk factors for first trimester miscarriage—results from a UK-population-based case-control study. *BJOG: An International Journal of Obstetrics and Gynaecology* 114:170–186.

Nackers, L. M., et al. 2010. The association between rate of initial weight loss and long-term success in obesity treatment: does slow and steady win the race? *International Journal of Behavioral Medicine* 17:161–167.

Nowson, C. A., 2003. Dietary approaches to reduce blood pressure in a community setting: a randomised crossover study. *Asia Pacific Journal of Clinical Nutrition* 12 Suppl:S19.

Rudkowska, I., et al. 2008. Cholesterol-lowering efficacy of plant sterols in low-fat yogurt consumed as a snack or with a meal. *Journal of the American College of Nutrition* 27:588–595.

Sheets, V., and Ajmere, K. 2005. Are romantic partners a source of college students' weight concern? *Eating Behaviors* 6:1–9.

Tran, T. T. 2008. Beneficial effects of subcutaneous fat transplantation on metabolism. *Cell Metabolism* 7:410–420.

Chapter 2: Burn, Baby, Burn

Beil, L. 2010. Fat chance: scientists are working out ways to rev up the body's gut-busting machinery. *Science News*, July 3 issue.

Diamant, M., 2010. Do nutrient-gut-microbiota interactions play a role in human obesity, insulin resistance and type 2 diabetes? *Obesity Review*, August 13.

Editor. 2003. Vegetarian today: yogurt is a smooth substitute. *South Florida Sun-Sentinel*. September 11.

Kim, D. H., et al. 2010. Peptide designed to elicit apoptosis in adipose tissue endothelium reduces food intake and body weight. *Diabetes* 59:907–915.

Lyons, C. 1999. Water: drink to your health. *Ebony*, July.

McCrory, M. A., et al. 1999. Dietary variety within food groups: association with energy intake and body fatness in men and women. *American Journal of Clinical Nutrition* 69:440–447.

Norvell, C. 1996. Yogurt: a wealth of benefits. *Better Nutrition*, May.

Pataky, Z. 2009 Gut microbiota, responsible for our body weight? *Revue Medicale Suisse* 5:662–664, 666.

Scarpellini, E. 2010. Gut microbiota and obesity. *Internal and Emergency Medicine* 5 Supplement 1:S53–56.

Siple, M. 2006. Detox without fasting: need a spring cleanse, but don't want to go hungry? *Natural Health*, April.

Yang, C. S., and Wang, X. 2010. Green tea and cancer prevention. *Nutrition and Cancer* 62(7):931–937.

Chapter 3: Contour Foods: Nutritional Spot Reduction

Aceto, C. 2009. "Principles of getting ripped: 20 nutritional tips for a leaner you. *Flex*, April.

Aller, E. E., et al. 2011.Starches, sugars and obesity. *Nutrients* 3:341–369.

Barbosa, J. C., et al. 1990. The relationship among adiposity, diet, and hormone concentrations in vegetarian and nonvegetarian postmenopausal women. *Journal of the American College of Clinical Nutrition* 51:798–803.

Boghossian, N. S., et al. 2013. Adherence to the Mediterranean diet and body fat distribution in reproductive aged women. *European Journal of Clinical Nutrition* 67:289–294.

Ryberg, M., et. al. 2013.A Palaeolithic-type diet causes strong tissue-specific effects on ectopic fat deposition in obese postmenopausal women. *Journal of Internal Medicine* 274:67–76.

Spencer M., et al. 2013. Omega-3 fatty acids reduce adipose tissue macrophages in human subjects with insulin resistance. *Diabetes* 62:1709–1717.

Thomas, D.T., et al. 2011. Effects of a dairy supplement and resistance training on lean mass and insulin-like growth factor in women. *International Journal of Sport Nutrition and Exercise Metabolism* 21:181–188.

Vergnaud, A. C., et al. 2008. Dairy consumption and 6-y changes in body weight and waist circumference in middle-aged French adults. *American Journal of Clinical Nutrition* 88:1248–1255.

Chapter 4: The Fasting Breakthrough

Baer, D. J., et. al. 2011. Whey protein but not soy protein supplementation alters body weight and composition in free-living overweight and obese adults. *Journal of Nutrition* 141:1489–1494.

Fukino, Y., et al. 2008. Randomized controlled trial for an effect of green tea-extract powder supplementation on glucose abnormalities. *European Journal of Clinical Nutrition* 62: 953–960.

Jakubowicz, D., and Froy, O. 2013. Biochemical and metabolic mechanisms by which dietary whey protein may combat obesity and Type 2 diabetes. *The Journal of Nutritional Biochemistry* 24:1–5.

McPherson, R. A., et al. 2011. Clinical and nutritional benefits of cysteine-enriched protein supplements. *Current Opinion in Clinical Nutrition and Metabolic Care* 14:562–568.

Sousa, G. T., et al. 2012. Dietary whey protein lessens several risk factors for metabolic diseases: a review. *Lipids in Health and Disease* 11:67.

Trepanowski, J. F., and Bloomer, R. J. 2010. The impact of religious fasting on human health. *Journal of Nutrition* 22: 57.

Weiss, D. J., and Anderton, C. R. 2003. Determination of catechins in matcha green tea by micellar electrokinetic chromatography. *Journal of Chromatography* 1011:173–180.

Zipes, D. 2003. Keeping fit with fiber. *Medical Update*, January Issue.

Chapter 5: Cycle 1: Accelerate

Aronson, D. 2002. 50 foods to help you look and feel great: these are your best choices to lose weight, boost your energy. *Natural Health*, March.

Charatan, J. 2000. Eat to your heart's content. *Vegetarian Times*, February.

Editor. 1999. Healthy eating. *Ebony*, July.

Gormley, J. J. 1999. Giving the liver some respect. *Better Nutrition*, December.

Simon, A. 1984. New angles on fish dishes. *Saturday Evening Post*, May-June.

Tremblay, A., et al. 2004. Thermogenesis and weight loss in obese individuals: a primary association with organochlorine pollution. *International Journal of Obesity and Related Metabolic Disorders* 28(7):936–939.

Chapter 6: Cycle 2: Activate

Aceto, C. 2002. Carbohydrate cycling: this seven-point diet strategy will help you keep bodyfat in check. *Flex*, October.

Jakulj, F. 2007. A high-fat meal increases cardiovascular reactivity to psychological stress in healthy young adults. *Journal of Nutrition* 137:935–939.

Liu, H. 2010. Fructose induces transketolase flux to promote pancreatic cancer growth. *Cancer Research* 70:6368–6376.

Varady, K.A. 2007. Alternate-day fasting and chronic disease prevention: a review of human and animal trials. *American Journal of Clinical Nutrition* 86:7–13.

Walsh, J. 1997. Choosing lean over not-so-lean beef and pork cuts. *Environmental Nutrition*, February.

Westerterp-Planteng, M.S., et al. 2005. Sensory and gastrointestinal satiety effects of capsaicin on food intake. *International Journal of Obesity* 29:682–688.

Chapter 7: Cycle 3: Achieve

Di Blasio, A. 2010. Effects of the time of day of walking on dietary behaviour, body composition and aerobic fitness in post-menopausal women. *The Journal of Sports Medicine and Physical Fitness* 50:196–201.

Fischer-Posovszky, P. 2010. Resveratrol regulates human adipocyte number and function in a Sirt1-dependent manner. *American Journal of Clinical Nutrition* 92:5–15.

Fuchs, N. K. 2002. Liposuction lowers cholesterol. *Women's Health Letter*. Soundview Publications, June 1.

Kristal, A. R. 2005. Yoga practice is associated with attenuated weight gain in healthy, middle-aged men and women. *Alternative Therapies in Health and Medicine* 11:28–33.

National Weight Control Registry. www.nwcr.ws/Research/default.htm.

Rolls, B. J., et al. 2004. Salad and satiety: energy density and portion size of a first-course salad affect energy intake at lunch. *Journal of the American Dietetic Association* 104:1570–1576.

Vgontzas, A. N. 2007. Daytime napping after a night of sleep loss decreases sleepiness, improves performance, and causes beneficial changes in cortisol and interleukin-6 secretion. *American Journal of Physiology, Endocrinology, and Metabolism* 292: E253–E261.

Chapter 8: Cycle 4: Arrive

Mermelstein, S. P. Weekends off. *Good Housekeeping*, January.

Henson, S. 2005. Cook light, cook right (weight matters). *Paraplegia News*, September issue.

Rebello, C. J., et al. 2013. Dietary strategies to increase satiety. *Advances in Food and Nutrition Research* 69:105–182.

Tallmadge, K. 2003. 15 simple tricks for lasting weight loss: lose 5–40 pounds (or more!) this year. *Shape*, January.

Chapter 9: The 17 Day Cultural Diet

Editor. 2009. Eat like the Greeks: by adopting a Mediterranean-style diet, you may help ward off heart disease. *Men's Health Advisor*, May.

Eller, D. 2004. The spices of life: here's a healthful and spiritual approach to vegetarian Indian cooking. *Natural Health*, April.

Francisco, J. 2006. Pasta sauce: ensure your hearty Italian dinner is a healthful one. *Better Nutrition*, February.

Louie, E. 2008. From an Iranian cook, the taste of memory. *The New York Times*, January 9.

Chapter 10: The PMS Exception Diet

Benton, D., and Cook, R. 1991. The impact of selenium supplementation on mood. *Biological Psychiatry* 29:1092–1098.

Editor. 2004. PMS breakthroughs: doctors now believe there are actually five different types of PMS. *Marie Claire*, June.

Ghanbari Z., et al. 2009 Effects of calcium supplement therapy in women with premenstrual syndrome. *Taiwan Journal Obstetrics and Gynecology* 48:124–129.

Grumman, R. 2006. Be the boss of your period: feeling fat, crampy, and cranky month after month after month is no way for a modern girl to live. *Cosmopolitan*, June.

Hawkes, W. C., and Hornbostel, L. 1996. Effects of dietary selenium on mood in healthy men living in a metabolic research unit. *Biological Psychiatry* 39:121–128.

Hibbeln, J. R. 1998. Fish consumption and major depression. *The Lancet* 351:1213.

Hibbeln, J. R., and Salem, N. 1995. Dietary polyunsaturated fatty acids and depression: when cholesterol does not satisfy. *American Journal of Clinical Nutrition* 62: 1–9.

Kalman, D., et al. 2009. A prospective, randomized, double-blind, placebo-controlled parallel-group dual site trial to evaluate the effects of a Bacillus coagulans-based product on functional intestinal gas symptoms. *BMC Gastroenterology* 18:85.

Smith, J. K. 1999. Eat to beat PMS. *Redbook*, April.

Turner, L. 2008. Chocolate: a love affair. *Better Nutrition*, February 1.

Wadyka, S. 2002. This is your PMS survival kit: is your period a pain? *Redbook*, June.

Chapter 11: Dining Out on the 17 Day Diet

Editor. 2007. Eating a single high-fat meal can raise blood pressure significantly more than a very low-fat meal. *Environmental Nutrition*, July.

Editor. 2002. Whale of a whopper: A lot of "good" restaurant food has got a lot of fat. *Philadelphia Daily News*. June 5.

Chapter 12: Family Challenges

Editor. 2009. Couples find success in losing weight together. *The Pittsburgh Tribune-Review*. October 13.

Morgan, D.V., et al. 1988. Mutual motivation. *Health*, August.

Paisley J., et al. 2008. Dietary change: what are the responses and roles of significant others? *Journal of Nutrition Education and Behavior* 40:80–88.

Stedman, Nancy. 1996. How to lose weight when you live with a man. *Redbook*, May.

Wallace, J. P. 1995. Twelve month adherence of adults who joined a fitness program with a spouse vs. without a spouse. *Journal of Sports Medicine and Physical Fitness* 35:206–213.

Chapter 13: Surviving Holidays

Andersson, I., et al. 1992. The Christmas factor in obesity therapy. *International Journal of Obesity and Related Metabolic Disorders* 16:1013–1015.

Baker, R. C. et al. Weight control during the holidays: Highly consistent self-monitoring as a potentially useful coping mechanism. *Health Psychology* 17:367–370.

Editor. 2005. Beating back the New Year's bulge: cheating away those holiday pounds. *PR Newswire*, December 20.

Editor. 2002. Turn holiday calories into muscle. *Men's Fitness*, November.

Fiedler, C. 2008. Stressed out? But here's the good news: the secret to staying healthy and feeling energized is simple. *Natural Health*, May.

Gordon, T. 2004. Keep the happy in your holidays: don't let stress, overindulgence, and sleep deficits spoil your fun. *Vibrant Life*. November-December.

Chapter 14: The 17 Day Diet on the Road

Bowie, D. 2005. Fit to work: there's no longer any excuse to be idle on your business trips. *Business Traveller Middle East*, May-June.

Editor. 2001. Planning lets you fit fitness into your travels. *The Orange County Register*, July 12 issue.

Galusha, D. E., and Holt, B. R. 2008. Frequent flyer, frequent pounds. *Vibrant Life*, Jan-Feb.

Chapter 15: Shift Work on the 17 Day Diet

Geliebter, A. 2000. Work-shift period and weight change. *Nutrition* 16:27–29.

Henderson, N. J., and Christopher D. B. B. 1998. An evaluation of the effectiveness of shift work preparation strategies. *New Zealand Journal of Psychology*. New Zealand Psychological Society 27: accessed on questia.com.

Johnson, C. 1999. Don't forget your shift workers. *HR Magazine*, February.

Kirn, T. F. 2006. Artificial lighting may play role in rising obesity rate. *Internal Medicine News*, December.

Thorpy, M. J. 2010. Managing the patient with shift-work disorder. *The Journal of Family Practice* 59(1 Suppl):S24–31.

Chapter 16: Supplement Sense on the 17 Day Diet

Challem, J. 2007. Minerals 101: vitamins usually grab the headlines, but dietary minerals are just as important. *Better Nutrition*, August.

Chen, S. C., et al. 2012. Effect of conjugated linoleic acid supplementation on weight loss and body fat composition in a Chinese population. *Nutrition* 28: 559–565.

Damms-Machado, A., et al. 2012. Micronutrient deficiency in obese subjects undergoing low calorie diet. *Nutrition Journal* 11:34.

Editor. 2009. Consumers and healthcare professionals agree: kitchen cabinet is home for my supplements. *US Newswire*, February 24.

Hanson, C. 2006. CLA: conjugated linoleic acid may help you shed those unwanted pounds you gained in 2005. Here's how. *Better Nutrition*, January.

Mandile, M. N. 2001. Federal panel pushes heart pills: the government claims prescriptions beat prevention when it comes. *Natural Health*, September.

Rosenblum. J. L., et al. 2012. Calcium and vitamin D supplementation is associated with decreased abdominal visceral adipose tissue in overweight and obese adults. *American Journal of Clinical Nutrition* 95: 101–108.

Chapter 17: The 17 Minute Spot Reduction Workout

Editor. 2005. Practice yoga, stay slim, healthy: American researchers. *The Press Trust of India Ltd.*, August 5.

Kerig, B. 1994. Weak in the knees?: building up muscles that support the knees. *Men's Health*, December.

Chapter 19: Mister M.D., Can You Please Tell Me More?

Atkinson, J. 2001. The funny thing about cholesterol: risks for heart disease and how cholesterol is affected. *Esquire*, June.

Checkoway H., et al. 2002. Parkinson's disease risks associated with cigarette smoking, alcohol consumption, and caffeine intake. *American Journal of Epidemiology*. 155:732–738.

Drayer, L. 2009. Are there foods I can eat for better skin? *Redbook*, March.

Editor. 2010. Ask the doctor. *Healthy Years*, February.

Editor. 2003. Ask the nutritionist. *Shape*, March.

Editor. 2010. An inside look at sugar substitutes. *Food & Fitness Advisor*, August.

Editor. 2007. Trying to quit smoking? Get moving. *Shape Magazine*, February 1.

Karolyn, A. G. 2008. Reversing prediabetes. *Better Nutrition*.

Marian, T. et al. 2000. Effect of dietary protein on bone loss in elderly men and women: The Framingham Osteoporosis Study. *Journal of Bone and Mineral Research* 15:2504–2512.

Shengxu L., et al. 2010. Physical activity attenuates the genetic predisposition to obesity in 20,000 men and women from EPIC-Norfolk prospective population study. *PLOS Medicine* e1000332. doi:10.1371/journal.pmed.1000332.

van Dam, R. M., et al. 2006. Coffee, caffeine, and risk of type 2 diabetes: a prospective cohort study in younger and middle-aged U.S. women. *Diabetes Care* 29:398–403.

About the Author

Dr. Michael Rafael Moreno, better known as Dr. Mike, is a graduate of the University of California at Irvine and Hahnemann Medical School (now Drexel University). Following his residency at Kaiser Permanente in Fontana, California, Dr. Mike moved to San Diego, where he now practices family medicine and sits on the board of the San Diego Chapter of the American Academy of Family Physicians.

In 2008, Dr. Mike launched "Walk with Your Doc" (http://www.walkwithyourdoc.com), which he participates in every Tuesday and Thursday morning before his work day begins. The program began when Dr. Mike offered to walk with a patient to motivate her to exercise, and has since grown into a thriving community.

Dr. Mike takes pride in being viewed not only as a doctor, but also as a friend and confidant.

"We've all pledged, promised, and bullied ourselves to eat better and exercise more, but so many times even the best intentions fall short," Dr. Mike says. "I incorporate healthy habits into my work and home life, and you can too."